# Advances in Mental Health and Addiction

## SpringerBriefs in Advances in Mental Health and Addiction

**Series Editor**

Masood Zangeneh, Richmond Hill, ON, Canada

W0234540

Over the past several decades we have witnessed dramatic shifts in prevailing approaches to mental health and addiction. Significant scientific achievements have led to novel treatment options that impacted the experiences of individuals with mental disorders. In recent years, new perspectives have begun to influence the way we address mental health and substance dependencies, resulting in a greater emphasis on mental health promotion and prevention strategies. Despite these progressions, mental health care systems too often remain stagnant, fragmented, and peripheral.

Masood Zangeneh

Humber College, Woodbridge, ON, Canada

This sub-series provides an opportunity to expand upon cutting-edge research being presented at mental health or addiction related conferences or colloquia around the world. Each 50-125 page volume would be dedicated to a singular event and would provide an opportunity for scholars to present their research and get feedback from other scholars in their field.

Dionisio Nyaga • Rose Ann Torres

Editors

# Reimagining Mental Health and Addiction Under the Covid-19 Pandemic, *Volume 1*

The Covid-19 Pandemic, Mental Health, and Ethnicity

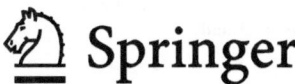 Springer

*Editors*
Dionisio Nyaga
Algoma University
Sault Ste. Marie, ON, Canada

Rose Ann Torres
Algoma University
Sault Ste. Marie, ON, Canada

ISSN 2570-3390          ISSN 2570-3404   (electronic)
Advances in Mental Health and Addiction
ISSN 2948-2224          ISSN 2948-2232   (electronic)
SpringerBriefs in Advances in Mental Health and Addiction
ISBN 978-3-031-58366-7          ISBN 978-3-031-58367-4   (eBook)
https://doi.org/10.1007/978-3-031-58367-4

This Springer imprint is published by the registered company Springer Nature Switzerland AG
The registered company address is: Gewerbestrasse 11, 6330 Cham, Switzerland

If disposing of this product, please recycle the paper.

# Preface

This manuscript comes from a place of ethical nature of how we need to engage with community mental health, more especially during pandemic. The ground for this piece is based on experiences of marginalized communities and how they faced Covid-19. Covid 19 affected communities in unique ways. This piece therefore calls for a reimagination of how we work with pandemics to start another conversation that is beyond quantification and qualification of pandemics. This is the ethical background in the conceptualization of this book. This edited collection is a follow up to Algoma University inaugural International Conference on Mental Health and Addiction held in Brampton campus Ontario Canada in April 2023. The conference brought diverse stakeholders on this special topic and was widely attended by mental health practitioners, researchers, and community organizations from across the world. The focus was to look at how Covid-19 had compounded community mental health based on the ways in which communities continued to face the pandemic in unique ways. The conference has diverse ways of approaching the pandemic and they all converged on the question of how we could approach future pandemics based on the lesson learned from Covid-19. It became clear that the pandemic has clearly opened avenues of understanding mental health beyond the current quantitative and simplistic metric. Questions of historical events, values, and realities of people became the central binding thread in imagining what communities and other stakeholders were facing during and after the pandemic.

We live in a society wherein many marginalized communities among them Black, Brown, Indigenous, Queer and Trans individuals, and many others continue to face historically difficult and disproportionate weight on their psychological, mental, and economic well-being more so under the Covid-19 pandemic. Covid-19 continues to affect marginalized/minorities, racialized communities in all levels. We now see the compounded impacts in the forms of the latest escalating mental health and addiction crisis and the subsequent effect that has on education among the children, service delivery, and overall psychosocial well-being. Covid-19 widened the gap and poverty between high- and low-income people, and more than that it affects the psychosocial resilience of the people. As communities of scholars, practitioners, and researchers, we owe it to our communities to engage with these existential issues in ways that are ethical and transformative. This form of engagement should help ameliorate the consequences of the pandemic in ways that are intersectional. Such conversations should help us come to terms and engage with the trauma and pain that marginalized communities and people continue to face and how we can work together to 'find' answers toward addressing issues of mental health and addiction. We need to value people's histories and realities in their intersectional engagement to bring forth a form of social justice that goes beyond treatments of mental health and addiction.

Black, Indigenous, Asian, and other marginalized communities have faced the pandemic in ways that continue to affect their mental health and addiction in disproportionate ways (Gaynor & Wilson, 2020; Tamagawa, 2023; Zhai et al., 2023). This means that on top of prevailing historical colonial trauma in Canada (Walker, 2008), these communities must work more toward healing from the impact of Covid-19 on their mental health and addiction. On top of that, we are now being invited to prepare ourselves for a world that is pandemic. While most marginalized communities will have to contend with what happened before and during the Covid-19 pandemic, they will now have to imagine new ways of living with future pandemics. This is not only challenging but also provides an opportunity to employ new ways of coping with pandemics in ways that are not only quantitative but ethically responsible. This means our efforts to curb future pandemics as suggested by the World Health Organization are limited if we fail to consider the histories, values, and realities of the most marginalized communities. In this regard, a new methodology of approving scientific measures of curbing future pandemics needs to be centered toward meeting the holistic socio-cultural and economic health of communities in the age of pandemics. This will ensure that not only do we deal with curbing the spread of the current and future pandemics, but we do that in ways that are ethical, balanced, and sustainable.

Jodi Webber's chapter looks at re-evaluating identity theories to reflect changing circumstances of care providers. The chapter argues that with the Covid-19 pandemic and its aftermath, it is ethically possible to rethink caregiving in ways that help bring justice to care givers. Elisha Denise et al. look at the ways in which families coped with the death of their loved one during the Covid-19 pandemic. The question of social and physical distance as a measure to curb the spread of Covid-19 affected how people buried their loved one, thus compounding their mental health. How then could communities care for the dead during the pandemic and how would such a community reconcile the failure to be present for their dead loved one? Gabrielle (Bulahan) et al. look at the experiences of Filipino queer students and how they navigate the politics of the cabinet. This piece opens complexities of identity politics and consequently critiquing representational politics that guide a heteronormative society. April Mae et al. look at the consequences of climate change on communities living in the Philippines and calls for a concerted effort to educate and sensitize communities on the same. Meghan et al. look at how Covid-19 affected field office in social work sector. This topic is an important one since much was and has never been discussed on how social work practicum was affected by Covid-19. Tanya and Allyson Theodorou looks at the effect of the Covid-19 pandemic in service provision and ways in which such lessons have implication in providing care that is ethical and political.

Sidney Wilson looks at challenges of teaching and learning more so with children who face mental health. This chapter helps reimagine school system in ways that are open to student diverse needs. Judy Rebek et al. investigate the transformative power of Meditative Inquiry (MI) during the Covid-19 pandemic in higher education. This mixed method study helps reimagine social life in ways that are transformative and ethical. Teryn Bruni looks at how post-Covid-19 could continue affecting teaching and learning and why as educators we need to pay attention to this academic gap. Bruni seeks to reimagine the curriculum in ways that are ethically possible for both the educator and the learner. Fritz Pino's chapter introduced us to the limitation of current mental health discourse more so to Filipino queer and trans communities. The chapter calls for re-imagination of mental health care in ways that are ethical and grounded in transformative change.

Rose Ann Torres, Valerie Damasco, Aprilyn Encina Calvario, and Yashoda Fernando pay attention to care giving amid Covid-19 and how that affected Filipino nurses. The chapter looks at the strength of caregivers amid the Covid-19 pandemic to start asking ethical questions on differentiated care giving technologies. Maryam Motia's chapter looks at the changes of mental health accessibility among immigrant communities and calls for reimagination of mental health discourse to start open spaces for immigrant populations.

Sault Ste. Marie, ON, Canada

Dionisio Nyaga
Rose Ann Torres

# References

Gaynor, T. S., & Wilson, M. E. (2020). Social vulnerability and equity: The disproportionate impact of COVID-19. *Public Administration Review, 80*(5), 832–838. https://doi.org/10.1111/puar.13264

Tamagawa, M. (2023). *The Japanese LGBTQ+ community in the world: The COVID-19 pandemic, challenges, and prospects for the future.* Routledge, Taylor & Francis Group.

Walker, B. (2008). *The history of immigration and racism in Canada: Essential readings* (B. Walker, Ed.).Canadian Scholars' Press

Zhai, W., Fu, X., Liu, M., & Peng, Z.-R. (2023). The impact of ethnic segregation on neighbourhood-level social distancing in the United States amid the early outbreak of COVID-19. *Urban Studies, 60*(8), 1403–1426. https://doi.org/10.1177/00420980211050183

# Acknowledgments

We would like to acknowledge the work of so many people who have been persistent in making sure these discussions are made public. First, we acknowledge several people who found time to organize the Algoma University international conference on mental health and addiction. Several people are worth mentioning. These are Dr. Suleyman Demi, Dr. Deb Woodman, Dr. Fritz Pino, Meghan Boston McCracken, and so many others who took time out of their busy schedule to make the conference a success. It was outside of that conference that we found ourselves engaged in a book project of this magnitude. We also want to thank those who found time to contribute to this project that comes at a point where many edged out communities faced the Covid-19 pandemic in ways that were compounded and unique. Thanks for finding time to bring your contribution to this project. We appreciate your time and your dedication to making this project a success.

# Contents

# Understanding the Mental Health Experiences of Unpaid Caregivers: The Role and Limitations of Caregiver Identity Theory

Jodi Webber

## Introduction

The COVID-19 pandemic disrupted already fragile support networks for older adults and their unpaid family and friend caregivers. With healthcare systems overwhelmed and restrictions on accessing support services, caregivers had to take on additional responsibilities (Canadian Centre for Caregiving Excellence, 2022). These increased care demands, along with social isolation and the overall uncertainty and stress of the pandemic negatively impacted the mental health and well-being of caregivers (Chiu et al., 2022; Irani et al., 2021; Leggett et al., 2022; Truskinovsky et al., 2022). Caregivers reported increased rates of depression and anxiety, not only threatening the overall health of the caregivers (Boyd et al., 2022) but challenging their ability to continue providing care. In Canada this represents an estimated $9.71 billion annually in unpaid care work to older people, people living with disabilities, and people with functional limitations (Eales et al., 2022). The care economy is 4.2% of our GDP (Eales et al., 2022). Caregivers must have better support.

With the field of social work committed to the principles of equity, diversity, and inclusion across all levels of practice, there has never been a better time to examine the theories regularly used to interpret and analyse our work. Theory has an important role to play in understanding the mental health experiences of caregivers. Having a broad literature base drawn across many disciplinary traditions helps us to conceptualize caregiving, predict caregiver distress, and design evidence-based interventions and programmes that aim to socially support caregivers, provide education, and offer respite. Theory-based research also has a role in informing public

J. Webber (✉)
School of Social Work, Algoma University, Sault ste Marie, ON, Canada
e-mail: jodi.webber@algomau.ca

© The Author(s), under exclusive license to Springer Nature Switzerland AG 2024
D. Nyaga, R. A. Torres (eds.), *Reimagining Mental Health and Addiction Under the Covid-19 Pandemic*, Volume 1, Advances in Mental Health and Addiction,
https://doi.org/10.1007/978-3-031-58367-4_1

policy. The purpose of this chapter is to present a critique of the theory I apply most frequently in my work with unpaid family and friend caregivers, which is caregiver identity theory (Montgomery & Kosloski, 2009).

## Theoretical Overview

Caregiver identity theory (CIT) has made a considerable contribution to the field of caregiving research and approaches the caregiver experience from a role and identity lens. CIT offers a way of understanding the social construction of becoming a caregiver. There are three central tenets to the theory. According to Montgomery and Kosloski (2009), first, the caregiver role is acquired in a systematic way. Second, it is a dynamic process. And, third, assuming the role of caregiver changes the primary role. This theory posits that the caregiver role typically emerges from a primary familial role—usually spouse, child, or sibling. The evolution of the role, often understood as role conflict, challenges the ability to fulfil competing role obligations (spouse, parent, employee), creating tension (Montgomery & Kosloski, 2009). CIT assumes that the caregiving experience is highly unique and individualized, influenced by factors such as cultural background, socioeconomic status, and personal characteristics.

Based on CIT, the metamorphosis of the new identity happens in tandem with the care continuum. As the care recipient's needs change and increase over time, the role of caregiving dramatically extends or engulfs the previous role. Distress and strain typically occur when there is incongruence between the primary role and the new identity (Montgomery & Kosloski, 2009). There are many ways to conceptualize the role shift. Eifert et al. (2015), in their literature review of caregiver identity, identified "role engulfment and losing self, loss of shared identity, family obligation and gender norming, extension of the former role, and development of a master identity" as the most cited conceptualization of role shift (p. 364), each of these contributing to and shaping how the role of caregiver is defined and experienced.

Within CIT, the family rules, rituals, and boundaries (who is responsible for what) dictate the ease (or stress) of the transition (Segal et al., 2011). For example, in a heteronormative spousal relationship, perhaps the husband has been responsible for the grocery shopping, outside yard work and banking. According to CIT, role conflict arises when the wife is forced to take on these unfamiliar roles that subconsciously break the family's rules. Identity discrepancy is a significant source of distress, and reconciling the new caregiver role within the family system is important and challenging work (Montgomery et al., 2016).

Montgomery and Kosloski (2009) have conceptualized the progression of adopting the caregiving role as a five-phase process. Phase I is classified as the onset of the caregiving role, most likely defined by assistance with instrumental activities like banking and shopping. In this phase, the caregiver is unlikely to recognize the caregiver role. In Phase II, the caregiving role begins to extend beyond the usual familial identity, such as a daughter accompanying a parent to appointments, asking

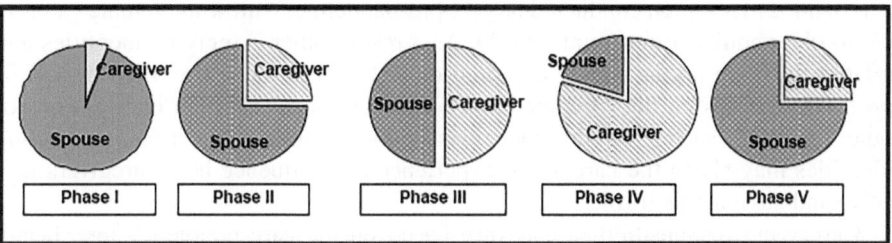

**Fig. 1** Phases of caregiver identity

the questions, and sharing information. Phase III is said to occur when the care needs of the recipient increase to the point where the caregiver identifies themself in the caregiver role and is struggling to straddle both identities. Phase IV is dominated by the caregiver role. At this point, the family may be contemplating long-term care. Phase V sees the return of the primary role as the major source of identity, as the recipient is institutionalized (Fig. 1).

Montgomery et al.' (2016) graphic representation of the phases of caregiver identity illustrates the experience of a spousal caregiver but is analogous to the example of the daughter as described in the main text. This figure is reproduced here with the permission of the Springer Publishing Company.

The strengths of CIT theory lie in its ability to guide practice with families. It provides a practical structure for health and social care providers to design and deliver timely services and supports for family caregivers. The phased approach depicted by Montgomery and Kosloski (2009) provides a visual cue that helps legitimize burden and distress. CIT also helps to explain distress and subsequently removes the blame the caregiver(s) may place upon themselves for the challenge or inability to cope.

Furthermore, research has typically focused on the caregiving experience from the lens of deficit. CIT however emphasizes the positive aspects of caregiving experiences. It recognizes that caregiving can provide opportunities for personal growth, purpose, and the development of valuable skills and attributes. The theory highlights the potential for caregiver identity development as a source of personal satisfaction and fulfilment.

## Limitations

We know the pandemic impacted caregivers in unforeseen ways, disrupting families and exacerbating distress (Boyd et al., 2022; Ontario Caregiver Organization, 2022; Truskinovsky et al., 2022), and as such, the limitations of CIT must be acknowledged. The empirical base of this approach could be strengthened. The theoretical foundations are underpinned by a gendered, Eurocentric, and heteronormative understanding of family and ageing, potentially limiting its applicability. The theory is grounded in research conducted largely pre-pandemic, with white female caregivers to older adults (Eifert et al., 2015). As a result, other caregiving identities and relationships are not as widely explored or included in the research schema. CIT primarily focuses on the caregiver's role without considering the intersections of other identities, such as gender, race, class, culture, and ability. These intersecting identities may shape the caregiving experience and influence how caregivers perceive and navigate their roles.

Caregiving responsibilities can vary based on the care recipient's age, health condition, and the availability of support systems (Eifert et al., 2015; Rurka et al., 2020). CIT does not explicitly address the impact of contextual factors on caregiver identity development. It would be valuable to have a greater understanding of caregiving needs across diseases, ages, and relationships for cross-comparison. This may provide the opportunity to develop a more tailored approach to support better health and well-being outcomes for caregivers through improved service use and increased help-seeking behaviour. Attention must turn to studying diverse family and caregiver partnerships to build our knowledge and policies. More diverse and inclusive streams of investigation may ultimately serve the Canadian healthcare system well.

The theory also assumes that caregiver identity development follows a linear process, whereby individuals progress from pre-caregiver to caregiver identity stages. Identity, however, is dynamic and does not necessarily follow the linear progression assumed by the theory. This again makes it more difficult to design interventions. As well, there are weak associations between care recipient needs and the caregiver's self-appraisal of commitment and responsibilities (Friedemann & Buckwalter, 2014). In fact, Montgomery and Kosloski (2013) conceded that appreciating which phase of the role a person is in provides little ability to successfully predict service needs.

The fifth phase is arguably problematic as it assumes that the transition back to the primary role is seamless; yet, despite being relieved of care responsibilities, many of the duties that shifted the role structure will remain permanent. Finally, it is worth considering that CIT would benefit from the inclusion of a sixth phase. Specifically, this final phase would incorporate the death of the care recipient, which has potential implications for the loss of both the caregiving role and the primary role. Eifert et al. (2015) point out that one can neither be a wife without a spouse, nor a child without a parent.

In conclusion, the spotlight on caregiving today suggests that there has never been a better time to reevaluate theories used to interpret the caregiver experience. The COVID-19 pandemic demonstrated that caregivers need better mental health supports if they are to remain resilient in their caring. As there is a burgeoning older adult population and a contraction of public services theories, they must broaden their understanding of identity, concepts of family, communities, and gender. Broadened theory has the potential to better inform practice and policy in more diverse and inclusive ways ultimately protecting the mental health of unpaid family and friend caregivers.

# References

Boyd, K., Winslow, V., Borson, S., Lindau, S. T., & Makelarski, J. A. (2022). Caregiving in a pandemic: Health-related socioeconomic vulnerabilities among women caregivers early in the COVID-19 pandemic. *Annals of Family Medicine, 20*(5), 406–413. https://doi.org/10.1370/afm.2845

Canadian Centre for Caregiving Excellence. (2022). *Giving care: An approach to a better caregiving landscape in Canada.* A. Foundation. https://canadiancaregiving.org/wp-content/uploads/2022/11/CCCE_Giving-Care.pdf

Chiu, M. Y. L., Leung, C. L. K., Li, B. K. K., Yeung, D., & Lo, T. W. (2022). Family caregiving during the COVID-19 pandemic: Factors associated with anxiety and depression of carers for community-dwelling older adults in Hong Kong. *BMC Geriatrics, 22*(1), 125. https://doi.org/10.1186/s12877-021-02741-6

Eales, J., Fast, J., Duncan, K., & Keating, N. (2022). *Value of family caregiving in Canada.* Research on Aging, Policies and Practice, University of Alberta. Retrieved July 29 from https://rapp.ualberta.ca/wp-content/uploads/sites/49/2022/02/Family-caregiving-worth-97-billion_2022-02-20.pdf

Eifert, E. K., Adams, R., Dudley, W., & Perko, M. (2015). Family caregiver identity: A literature review. *American Journal of Health Education, 46*(6), 357–367. https://doi.org/10.1080/19325037.2015.1099482

Friedemann, M.-L., & Buckwalter, K. C. (2014). Family caregiver role and burden related to gender and family relationships. *Journal of Family Nursing, 20*(3), 313–336. https://doi.org/10.1177/1074840714532715

Irani, E., Niyomyart, A., & Hickman, R. L., Jr. (2021). Family caregivers' experiences and changes in caregiving tasks during the COVID-19 pandemic. *Clinical Nursing Research, 30*(7), 1088–1097. https://doi.org/10.1177/10547738211014211

Leggett, A., Koo, H. J., Park, B., & Choi, H. (2022). The changing tides of caregiving during the COVID-19 pandemic: How decreasing and increasing care provision relates to caregiver well-being. *Journals of Gerontology: Series B, 77*(Supplement), S86–s97. https://doi.org/10.1093/geronb/gbac002

Montgomery, R. J. V., & Kosloski, K. (2009). Caregiving as a process of changing identity: Implications for caregiver support. *Generations: Journal of the American Society on Aging, 33*(1), 47–52. https://www.jstor.org/stable/26555632

Montgomery, R. J. V., & Kosloski, K. (2013). Pathways to caregiver identity and implications for support services. In R. J. V. Montgomery & R. C. Talley (Eds.), *Caregiving across the lifespan: Research, practice, policy* (pp. 131–156). Springer.

Montgomery, R. J. V., Kwak, J., & Kosloski, K. D. (2016). Theories guiding support services for family caregivers. In V. L. Bengtson & R. A. Settersten Jr. (Eds.), *Handbook of theories of aging* (3rd ed., pp. 443–462). Springer.

Ontario Caregiver Organization. (2022). *Spotlight report: Caregiving in year 3 of the pandemic.* https://ontariocaregiver.ca/wp-content/uploads/2022/12/OCO-Spotlight-Report-English-Final.pdf

Rurka, M., Suitor, J., & Gilligan, M. (2020). The caregiver identity in context: Consequences of identity threat from siblings. *The Journals of Gerontology: Series B.* https://doi.org/10.1093/geronb/gbaa099

Segal, D. L., Qualls, S. H., & Smyer, M. A. (2011). *Aging and mental health* (2nd ed.). Wiley-Blackwell.

Truskinovsky, Y., Finlay, J. M., & Kobayashi, L. C. (2022). Caregiving in a pandemic: COVID-19 and the well-being of family caregivers 55+ in the United States. *Medical Care Research and Review, 79*(5), 663–675. https://doi.org/10.1177/10775587211062405

# No See, No Touch: Coping Strategies Focused on Bereaved Family Members' Lived Experiences During the COVID-19 Pandemic

Elisha Denise A. Afloro, Aprilyn E. Calvario, Vianca Stephanie P. Basco, Neil Ryan S. Derla, Gio Manuel C. Garcia, Sharmaine B. Koh, and Precious C. Manguerra

## Introduction

The COVID-19 pandemic has had a significant impact on the mental health and well-being of family members who had unique experiences of losing and grieving for someone due to the health protocols imposed by the government. This health protocols had been reported to disrupt the grieving process of the bereaved family members negatively affecting their emotional, psychological, and social well-being (van Schaik et al., 2022).

A number of studies have explored the experiences people undergo when losing love ones. Yasgur (2021) discussed the the many grieving complexes and grieving process experienced by the bereaved family members focusing on how they deal with the loss. Torrens-Burton et al. (2022) argues that the disruption in the grieving process often leads to grieving even after death which could be due to unresolved emotions, a lack of closure, or the inability to fully process the loss due to the imposed limitations. This is the area that the study was looking for because of the many traditions that have constrained the bereaved family's chances to mourn.

This study aims to determine whether the coping methods of the bereaved family members in the Philippines differ from those in other nations.

Eventually, everything comes to an end, whether it does so in a positive or negative way. There is a need to find out if Zhai and Du's (2020) recommendation can be

E. D. A. Afloro · A. E. Calvario (✉) · V. S. P. Basco · N. R. S. Derla · G. M. C. Garcia · S. B. Koh · P. C. Manguerra
Polytechnic University of the Philippines Santa Rosa Laguna Campus, City of Santa Rosa, Laguna, Philippines
e-mail: edaafloro@iskolarngbayan.pup.edu.ph; aecalvario@pup.edu.ph; vspbasco@iskolarngbayan.pup.edu.ph; nrsderla@iskolarngbayan.pup.edu.ph; gmcgarcia@iskolarngbayan.pup.edu.ph; sbkoh@iskolarngbayan.pup.edu.ph; pcmanguerra@iskolarngbayan.pup.edu.ph

© The Author(s), under exclusive license to Springer Nature Switzerland AG 2024
D. Nyaga, R. A. Torres (eds.), *Reimagining Mental Health and Addiction Under the Covid-19 Pandemic,* Volume 1, Advances in Mental Health and Addiction, https://doi.org/10.1007/978-3-031-58367-4_2

adapted to Filipino culture. In their journal, they listed four strategies: choosing loss adaptation over loss coping, investigating and using adaptive strategies that will fit the bereaved person's personality and various situations, enabling the bereaved to continuously adjust to changes, and using self-efficacy and social support as tools to equip grievers with the ability to adapt to disruptions in the grieving process. Zhai and Du (2020) described the unique experiences people encountered in time of loss and grief during the COVID-19 pandemic. They suggested for a tailored and functional strategies to overcoming loss and grief to protect people's metal health and well-being during this unique experience. According to Walsh's (2020), therapists can effectively use the family resilience framework to assist families in building resilience in the face of the many difficulties they encounter and losses caused by the pandemic.

The study's theoretical basis draws from "Kapwa Theory" by Virgilio G. Enriquez and Bayanihan Spirit (1992) and "Bahala Na" by Senator Leticia Ramos-Shahani to understand how Filipino family members cope with the loss of a loved one during the COVID-19 pandemic. The term "kapwa" refers to the shared identity or inner self of individuals in Filipino culture. Enriquez proposed that understanding oneself involves recognizing the interconnectedness with others, emphasizing the importance of relationships and social harmony. The "Bayanihan Spirit," deeply rooted in Filipino culture, exemplifies communal unity and cooperation, where neighbors come together to assist one another in times of need. This tradition symbolizes the Filipino value of unity and collective action (Task Force on a Moral Recovery Program, 1988). "Bahala Na" reflects a cultural attitude of acceptance and surrender to fate or a higher power. It embodies resilience and trust in the face of uncertainty, reflecting the Filipino way of coping with adversity (Enriquez, 1992). This theoretical framework emphasizes the communal grieving process, practical support, and coping strategies as interconnected and essential components in the bereavement process of Filipino families during the pandemic's restricted burial protocols.

## *Research Design/Method*

In this study, a phenomenological type of qualitative research was employed to explore the experiences and coping strategies of bereaved family members during the COVID-19 pandemic. The study design was nonnumerical and used validated self-made guide questions to gather information, which was then organized into themes to draw conclusions and recommendations. Utilizing Moustakas' (1994) approach to transcendental phenomenology, the study investigated the coping strategies of family members during the implementation of strict burial protocol in the Philippines during Covid-19. According to Creswell and Creswell (2018), phenomenology aims to capture the universal essence of the lived experiences of individuals experiencing the same phenomenon.

## *Participants*

The study utilized convenience sampling to recruit 10 participants, consisting of 5 young adults and 5 adults aged 19 - 60 years old. Informed consent was given during the interviews. The participants were informed of the option to decline or discontinue their participation at any time during the conduct of the study.

Interviews was conducted either face-to-face or online and a written essay was sought from the participants. Consent and ethical considerations were sought from the participants. A psychological assistance was also provided in case the participants needed help in processing his or her emotions especially during the interview.

After all the data were collected, the researchers underwent debriefing, an opportunity for them to process their emotions, identify and address any ethical and personal issues that may have arisen during the interview process.

## *Data Analysis*

The study relied on the narratives obtained through in-depth interviews and from the written essays of the participants. The narratives were transcribed and coded for themes. Guided by the transcendental analysis process, the data were subjected to bracketing, horizontalization, theme clustering, textural descriptions leading to the essence of the study.

## *Research Instruments*

A researcher-made questionnaires were designed to elicit experiences and coping strategies from participants who lost a family member during Covid-19 pandemic when strict burial protocols were implemented. The questionnaires were reviewed by experts in psychology and qualitative research. It was also translated in Filipino language by a linguistic professor. This was done to cater to a diverse demographic profile of the selected participants to ensure that all questions were understood.

The researchers in this study ensured ethical principles were followed by obtaining approval from the university before conducting research. Informed consent was given during the interviews, and the language used was understandable to the participants. Participants were given the option to decline or discontinue their participation, and a disclaimer on data privacy was provided. A debriefing was given after informed consent, and the researchers corrected any misconceptions and provided appropriate information about the research. Additionally, the researchers followed the APA reference style and did not present the work or data of others as their own.

# Results and Discussion

## *Bracketing*

The researchers explored the experiences of bereaved family members during the COVID-19 pandemic. Though their backgrounds varied, they all shared the challenge of losing loved ones. Their stories included the loss of a best friend, a pet, physical contact with a mother, a daughter's disappearance, family members' COVID-19 infections, and the death of a grandmother. All the researchers faced emotions of sadness, yearning, and helplessness due to COVID-19 restrictions. They coped in different ways, such as relying on their faith, family, or determination. The researchers acknowledged their subjectivity and the need to reflect on how it might have influenced their analysis.

## *Horizontalization*

Researchers compiled a list of significant statements from participants on coping with the loss of loved ones during COVID-19 burials. The statements, divided into textural and structural categories, are shown in Table 1 and reflect common experiences among participants.

## *Theme Clustering*

The 78 significant statements of bereaved family members who experienced strict burial protocol during the COVID-19 pandemic were clustered into themes. The themes were utilized to answer the three research questions that shed light on the essence of the lived experience of the participants in the loss of their loved ones due to COVID-19 with restricted burial protocol (Table 2).

1. The Participants' Struggles as They Bereaved to the Loss of Their Loved Ones due to COVID-19 with Restricted Burial Protocol.

### Theme 1: *Unknown Farewell*

The COVID-19 pandemic has resulted to many challenges on individuals and families who lost a loved one. The theme, Unknown Farewell emerged as a prevalent concern among the participants who expressed that the pandemic has made the bereavement process particularly difficult and unnatural. The restrictions put in

**Table 1** Significance statements of bereaved family members lived experiences in their coping strategies for the loss of their loved one during strict burial protocols due to COVID-19 pandemic

| *Significant Statements* | |
| --- | --- |
| 1. the responsibility of being careful | 39. keeping oneself busy |
| 2. traveling required a number of documents to be processed | 40. drinking alcoholic drink as a way to vent out with family and friends |
| 3. limited number of family to attend | 41. cried and cried until fell asleep |
| 4. permitted to mourn for a day only | 42. use jokes and sense of humor |
| 5. too many restrictions | 43. praying |
| 6. inability to say goodbye, touch, or hug | 44. visiting the cemetery |
| 7. unable to see them alive or their body | 45. to accept that everyone will die |
| 8. came back as an ash | 46. loss is a natural part of life |
| 9. uncomfortable and disturbed sleep | 47. finding ways to move forward |
| 10. unable to focus on work | 48. support from oneself |
| 11. perplexed | 49. rational in the face of difficulties |
| 12. it happened so suddenly | 50. finding strength in adopting a mindset of resilience and determination |
| 13. difficulty adjusting to familiar routines and activities | 51. choosing to move forward memories of a loved one as motivation and inspiration to keep going |
| 14. cannot bond with them anymore | 52. able to think about good memories and feel positive emotions |
| 15. not seeing your loved one forever | 53. God has a plan for all of us |
| 16. difficulty finding a sense of normality and acceptance | 54. The Lord is good. |
| 17. cannot go outside | 55. death loved ones are in a better place |
| 18. cannot see anyone | 56. faith in the Lord |
| 19. isolated and unable to embrace each other. | 57. to continue life for the family |
| 20. harder to find support and closure in the grieving process | 58. to move forward |
| 21. last minute of the wake was forbidden | 59. continue and to look forward with life. |
| 22. desire to give proper burial | 60. able to share the situation |
| 23. desire to see the dead body of their loved ones as it was buried | 61. morally |
| 24. restrained | 62. financial |
| 25. catch a basin of heavy emotions in their family. | 63. received a lot of love |
| 26. solely rely on their own | 64. prayers |
| 27. asking God for strength | 65. appreciating the empathy and understanding |
| 28. lack of comfort | 66. makes you feel you are not alone. |
| 29. feeling of lost | 67. to continue life as what you have learned from your loss loved one |
| 30. feeling of emptiness | 68. knowing that your loss loved one is proud of you as you cope up with their loss |
| 31. remorse of unable to bond in the past | 69. focus more in fulfilling their dead loved ones' wishes |
| 32. couldn't fulfill promises | 70. gradually still in the process. |
| 33. mixed emotions towards different issues | 71. unknown feeling whether you had cope up or not |
| 34. wanted to cry | 72. can never adjust to the death |
| 35. emotional struggle | 73. devastating to know they are dead and cremated |
| 36. won't even think of yourself. | 74. time cannot really tell to move on |
| 37. a need to show strength | 75. gap in their heart. |
| 38. heartbroken, sad, angry, regret, and a lot more | 76. longingness in their heart. |
| | 77. have a feeling of waiting |
| | 78. things that triggers to remember their loved ones |

place to combat the spread of the virus have hindered the possibility of saying farewell nor visiting a loved one to pay respect for the last time. A related findings was reported by Becqué et al. (2021) stating that people struggled with the suddenness and unexpectedness of the pandemic and the resulting restricted burial protocols which can be described as unique and unnatural.

**Table 2** Theme clusters divided into six groups

| Theme Clusters | |
|---|---|
| **I. Textural Theme** | **II. Structural Theme** |
| **Theme 1: Unknown Farewell** | **Theme 3: A Sense to Cope Up** |
| Sub-Theme 1.1: Restricted Family Physical Gathering | Sub-themes 3.1: Strengthening Oneself to Continue Life |
| Sub-Theme 1.2 Struggling with the Absence of a Loved One | Sub-Theme 3.2: Acceptance of Death |
| Sub-Theme 1.3: Physiological Manifestation | Sub-Theme 3.3: Trust in God's Process |
| | **Theme 4: Importance of Surrounding Environment** |
| Sub-Theme 1.4: Limitations to Give Comfort | Sub-Theme 4.1: Family as a Source of Strength |
| **Theme 2: Emotional Roller Coaster Comes with Grieving** | Sub-Theme 4.2: Comfort from the External Support |
| Sub-Theme 2.1: Helplessness | **Theme 5: An Urge to Fulfill the Wishes of a Deceased Loved One** |
| Sub-Theme 2.2: Frustration | |
| Sub-Theme 2.3: Regulations of Emotions | **Theme 6: Uncertainty** |

### 1.1: Restricted Family Physical Gathering

The COVID-19 pandemic has made funeral practices and grieving process more difficult for many individuals. Participants reported feeling distressed by the restrictions that prevented them from visiting their loved ones in the chapel of rest or funeral homes such as travel ban, social distancing and stay-at-home orders. These restrictions caused further upset for family members which made the grieving process more difficult and painful.

### 1.2: Struggling with the Absence of a Loved One

The participants in the study struggled with the absence of their loved ones due to the suddenness of their loss, the lack of time to prepare and the difficulty accepting the finality of death. This experience of loss and grief left a void that was difficult for participants to fill, resulting to a struggle to come to terms with their new realities.

### 1.3: Physiological Manifestation

The sudden loss of a loved one during the pandemic has resulted to a range of physiological manifestations and emotional distress for many bereaved family members. The stress and grief brought by the pandemic have made it challenging for individuals to sleep and focus on their daily responsibilities, causing them further distress in their daily life activities.

### 1.4: Limitations to Give Comfort

The COVID-19 pandemic and associated restrictions has a profound impact on how people provided emotional and physical support to their loved ones during times of illness and death. The restrictions imposed to prevent the spread of virus made it difficult for people to physically be present with their grieving loved ones to offer comfort and sympathy. The absence of physical contact and face-to-face communication during funeral wakes and rites became challenging for participants. The new protocols restricted them to share their griefs and receive social support which are critical components in the grieving process. Just as what Cardoso et al. (2020) emphasized, "the exceptional regime determined by the pandemic abolished funerals and imposed necessary limitations on burials, creating disturbances rather than comforting" (p. 581).

### Theme 2: *Emotional Roller Coaster Comes with Grieving*

The participants experienced a multitude of emotions simultaneously and felt inundated by the intensity of their experiences. They reported experiencing feelings of anger, sadness, regret, and a range of other emotions. Additionally, the restrictions in place during that period exacerbated their sense of frustration and helplessness.

### 2.1: Helplessness

The COVID-19 pandemic and associated restrictions had a profound impact on the ability of family members to be present and offer support to their loved ones during times of illness and death. The lack of physical contact and inability to attend funerals and other end-of-life rituals created feelings of helplessness and despair for participants, who were unable to provide the support and comfort they would normally offer. The sense of being restrained and unable to connect with loved ones during their illness and death was a source of emotional distress, and participants reported feeling uncertain and lacking closure in the wake of their loved one's passing. This loss of control over events and the subsequent feeling of helplessness can trigger a range of emotions, including sadness, anger, and frustration.[2] Family members had to rely on their own support networks to navigate their grief, creating a "catch basin of heavy emotions" as they attempted to process their loss and manage their mental and emotional health.

### 2.2: Frustrations

The COVID-19 pandemic created significant challenges for those grieving the loss of loved ones. Participants reported feeling frustrated and overwhelmed by the physical separation from their loved ones during their final moments, which compounded the emotional distress of grief. The participants' inability to connect with the dying family members or loved ones through touch or direct eve contact deprived them of the opportunities to express compassion, gratitude, and love.

Participants also experienced feelings of guilt and remorse for not spending enough time with their loved ones and be able to talk to them during the final hour of a dying relative because of the health protocols imposed.

### 2.3: Regulations of Emotions
The lost of a loved one during the pandemic brought a range of emotions the participants had to deal with aside from coping with their own loss and grief. The participants had to continue with their jobs or work, look after the other family members who are also coping with the same loss and grief, and deal with their own sadness and grief over the loss of a family member. Coping with loss during a pandemic emphasized the different and unique challenges that the bereaved family members may have faced, as well as the pressures and responsibilities they may have felt.

2. *The Coping Strategies of the Bereaved Family Members as They Deal with the Death of Their Loved Ones due to the COVID-19 Pandemic with Restricted Burial Protocol.*

### Theme 3: *A Sense to Cope Up*

Bereaved participants in the study developed coping strategies to help them deal with the loss of their loved ones during the pandemic. They tried to be strong for themselves and accept that death is a natural part of life. Some participants also found comfort in their religious beliefs and rituals. This coping strategies were similar to the findings of Zavrou et al. (2022) that bereaved people often visit the grave of their loved ones and participate in religious activities to maintain a connection with the deceased and cope with their loss. These coping strategies also helped them establish a new bond with the deceased that was not traumatizing. By developing these coping strategies, participants were able to continue with their lives despite the painful loss of their loved ones.

### 3.1: Strengthening Oneself to Continue Life
Despite the challenges of losing loved ones during the pandemic, the participants resorted to various coping strategies to manage their grief such as keeping themselves busy or occupied with work or some activities, venting out with friends and family, frequent visiting of the deceased loved ones in the cemetery, and praying. This is similar to the findings of Segal et al. (2023) who reported that individuals cope with grief differently based on their life experiences and religious beliefs. Just like the participants, they have varied coping strategies deoending on what they deem relevant and useful.

## 3.2: Acceptance of Death

Based on the participants narratives, the acceptance of death is considered to be a personal decision and their strategies to overcome its pain is to find positive thoughts about it and reminisce precious memories of their loved ones. Wong (2017) identified three types of death acceptance: neutral acceptance, escape acceptance and approach acceptance. Some participants manifested neutral acceptance, recognizing death as a natural part of life while others demonstrated approach acceptance perceiving death as a bridge to the afterlife. Thus, participants showed death acceptance is a complex and personal process that can help people cope with grief and move forward in life.

## 3.3: Trust in God's Process

The participants in this study found solace in their faith and belief in the Divine plan which helped them cope with the loss of their loved ones. They were able to cope with the loss and at the same time strengthen their spirituality. In his article, Canete (2021) mentions that the Filipinos have very strong religious beliefs and this has helped them coped with the challenges brought by the COVID-19 pandemic.

## Theme 4: *Importance of Surrounding Environment*

Family and external support such as relatives, friends, and community are vital for the participants in coping with the loss of their loved ones. This support they have received helped them relieve their anguish, frustration, guilt, and such. Relieving their emotions helped them in internalizing their pain, also, validate, accept, and create a choice to move forward even if the load is too heavy to carry on.

## 4.1: The Family as a Source of Strength

Participants in the study recognized the significant role of family in coping with the loss of their loved ones. They looked at their families as their motivation and reasons to move on with their lives. The support they received from relatives provided them with a light of hope and a sense of purpose, enabling them to withstand and rebound from the adversity. For the participants, family resilience was considered a helpful coping and adaptation strategy in the face of loss and grief during COVID-19 pandemic. Thus being surrounded by their families as they grieved together was essential for the participants as they feel the support and empathy they needed in this unique grieving experience.

## 4.2: Comfort from External Support

The participants in the study identified external support, particularly from friends and church communities, as essential in coping with the loss of their loved ones during the pandemic. They were able to adjust to the situation and improve their well-being when they were surrounded by friends. Similarly, support from the community brought comfort and a positive outcome as they feel that many people were actually grieving with them. Chatter et al. (2015) discussed the that church-based support networks are effective in coping with life problems by providing concrete strategies and approaches to dealing with life problems and difficulties.

3. *The Lived Experiences of the Bereaved Family Members as They Employed Their Coping Strategies for the Death of their Loved Ones due to COVID-19 Pandemic with Restricted Burial Protocol.*

**Theme 5:** *An Urge to Fulfill the Wishes of a Deceased Loved One*

A coping strategy utilized by bereaved family members is to continue living their lives as their deceased loved ones would have expected them to. This belief helps fill the void of longingness experienced due to the loss of loved ones. By fulfilling their loved ones' wishes and aspirations, they found motivation to move forward and fulfill their own destinies. Even without the physical presence of their loved ones, the belief that they were still guiding and walking with them brought hope and aspiration. The death of their loved ones created a void in the participants' need for love, which was filled by their deceased loved ones. By fulfilling their loved ones' wishes, they hoped to fill the gap of loneliness and find satisfaction in achieving their loved ones' dreams for them. Ultimately, this belief allowed them to imagine that their loved ones' wishes and aspirations would live on forever through their actions.

**Theme 6:** *Uncertainty*

The death of a loved one is a difficult experience, and many participants expressed ambiguity in coping as they were unable to find closure. Thought they were able to adjust to the lost, uncertainty remained and the feeling of ambiguous loss persisted. The unresolved feelings of the participants were due to the lack of closure with their loved one because of the suddenness and the imposed restrictions. As Cormier, cited in Weir (2020) explained, when people are not physically present to bid goodbye and grieve with other mourners, they experience this feeling of ambiguity. The inability to have a funeral they wanted, offer prayers and songs, conduct religious rites or ceremonies contributed to this feeling of uncertainty.

## *Textural Description*

Themes 1 and 2 highlight the challenges faced by bereaved family members during restricted burial protocols. These emerging themes and sub-themes, such as unknown farewell and emotional roller coaster, shed light on the lived experiences of participants. The themes emphasize that grieving is a natural process, and restrictions on burial protocols can result in deeper losses beyond imagination. Participants struggle with limited physical gatherings and with absence, physiological manifestations, and limitations on giving comfort. Cultural burial practices provide comfort and warmth, but these are stripped away, causing helplessness, frustration, and challenges in regulating emotions. Despite understanding the pandemic situation, bereaved families lack compassion and warmth from the government, leading to a roller coaster ride of emotions.

## Structural Description

Themes 3, 4, 5, and 6 reveal four emerging themes and their sub-themes regarding how bereaved family members cope with the death of their loved ones, which address the second and third central questions of the research. The themes are A Sense to Cope Up, Importance of Surrounding Environment, An Urge to Fulfill the Wishes of a Deceased Loved One, and Uncertainty. The participants' coping strategies include strengthening oneself, accepting death, trusting in God's process, receiving support from family and friends, and fulfilling the wishes of their loved ones. While these strategies helped them during the strict burial protocol due to the COVID-19 pandemic and enabled them to find the motivation to continue embarking on their new lives, they still feel a void in their hearts. Some are experiencing ambiguous loss and still seek a sense of closure as they continue to move forward in their lives.

## Overall Essence

The core of the data under analysis in this study was connected through its theoretical basis, allowing researchers to examine the coping strategies and sentiments of participants who experienced restricted burial protocols during the COVID-19 pandemic. The study found that the coping strategies used by the participants were reflective of three Filipino cultural values and traits: the Kapwa Theory, Bayanihan Spirit, and Bahala Na attitude. These values emphasized interconnectedness, helping one another during times of need, and the acceptance of uncertainty and ability to cope with difficult situations.

Despite the standard safety precautions required during the pandemic, some participants still struggled with feelings of loss and difficulty in adjusting to their daily routine. The importance of the surrounding environment, such as family and external support, proved to be vital in providing strength and comfort to the bereaved family members.

The Bahala Na attitude was also evident among participants, as they coped with uncertainty and ambiguous loss due to the lack of a formal farewell. Nevertheless, the coping strategies they utilized, such as strengthening oneself, acceptance of death, trust in God's process, and fulfilling the wishes of the deceased, enabled them to be resilient in the face of adversity.

The "no see, no touch" phenomenon experienced by the participants was a double whammy of misfortune, not only stripping them of physical contact with their loved ones but also depriving them of the comforts that burial practices could provide. The rigid wake and burial protocols during the pandemic were beyond imagination, and the coping strategies used by the participants deserve acknowledgement for their resiliency.

This study highlights the importance of exploring the coping strategies used by individuals during devastating events to inform future studies, policies, and actions in mitigating disaster risk reduction management and palliative care.

## Discussion

This study explores the struggles of bereaved family members, their coping strategies, and how effective these strategies were during the COVID-19 pandemic's strict burial protocol. It explored the struggles of bereaved family members, their coping strategies, and how effective these strategies were during the COVID-19 pandemic's strict burial protocol. The goal was to provide valuable insights into the experiences of the bereaved and offer recommendations to improve disaster risk reduction management and palliative care for bereaved family members in future pandemics or disasters.

## Summary of Findings

1. As to the struggles of the bereaved family members.The study revealed two themes that highlighted the struggles of bereaved family members during the COVID-19 pandemic. Theme 1 centered around the unknown farewell experience, where physical gathering was restricted, and limitations to comfort were present, causing physiological and emotional manifestations. Sub-themes included struggling with the absence of a loved one and the burden of fastened health protocols. Theme 2 focused on the emotional roller coaster experienced by the participants, with sub-themes highlighting helplessness, frustration, and regulation of emotions. These findings shed light on the unconventional ways in which participants dealt with their emotions and the unprecedented loss of their loved ones during the pandemic.
2. As to how bereaved family members cope as they deal with the death of their loved ones.The study identified two emerging themes related to how bereaved family members cope with the death of their loved ones during the pandemic. Theme 3 explored the coping strategies chosen by the participants, including

strengthening oneself, acceptance of death, and trust in God's process. These coping strategies helped them move forward with their loss, although the pain and love remained. Theme 4 highlighted the importance of support from the participants' surrounding environment, including family, relatives, friends, and churchmates. The support they received was crucial in helping them cope with their loss.

3. As to how did the coping strategies employed by the family members help them during the strict burial protocol due to the COVID-19 pandemic.

4. The data analysis revealed two themes on how the coping strategies employed by family members helped them during the strict burial protocol due to the COVID-19 pandemic. Theme 5 highlighted the urge to fulfill the wishes of their deceased loved ones as a way of feeling reunited with them. By fulfilling these wishes, they filled the void of despair, frustration, and loneliness. On the other hand, Theme 6 focused on the uncertainty of the coping strategies they used to move forward after the death of their loved ones. They questioned whether they had truly moved on or just continued with life after the loss. These themes shed light on the complexities of grief and coping strategies, especially during unprecedented times like a pandemic.

## Conclusions

The researchers found that bereaved Filipino family members faced significant challenges and struggled with physical, physiological, and mental issues due to restricted burial protocols during the COVID-19 pandemic. However, the study also revealed that the coping strategies employed by these family members were rooted in a holistic approach that included practical support, communal grieving, and coping mechanisms such as acceptance of death and trust in God's process. The study's eclectic theoretical framework, which incorporated Kapwa Theory, Bayanihan Spirit, and Bahala Na attitude, provided a comprehensive understanding of these coping strategies. While it was unclear whether participants had moved on or simply moved forward after their loved one's death, their resilience during these difficult times was evident.

## Recommendations

Based on the results of the study, is it recommended that in the event of mourning for a loved one, the bereaved family members may be encouraged to seek emotional support and counseling to help them process their emotions... programs that offer counseling and support may be created and be made available to bereaved family members. Since the study is purely qualitative, it is suggested to conduct further investigation using quantitative and expand the demographics of the participants.

# References

Becqué, Y. N., van der Geugten, W., van der Heide, A., Korfage, I. J., Pasman, H. R. W., Onwuteaka-Philipsen, B. D., Zee, M., Witkamp, E., & Goossensen, A. (2021). Dignity reflections based on experiences of end-of-life care during the first wave of the COVID-19 pandemic: A qualitative inquiry among bereaved relatives in The Netherlands (the CO-LIVE study). *Scandinavian Journal of Caring Sciences, 36*(3), 769–781. https://doi.org/10.1111/scs.13038

Canete, J. J. O. (2021). When expressions of faith in The Philippines become a potential COVID-19 "superspreader". *Journal of Public Health, 43*(2), e366–e367. https://doi.org/10.1093/pubmed/fdab082

Cardoso, R. A. D. O., Silva, B. C. D. A. D., Santos, J. H. D., Lotério, L. D. S., Accoroni, A. G., & Santos, M. A. D. (2020). The effect of suppressing funeral rituals during the COVID-19 pandemic on bereaved families. *Revista Latino-Americana de Enfermagem, 28*. https://doi.org/10.1590/1518-8345.4519.3361

Chatters, L. M., Taylor, R. J., Woodward, A. T., & Nicklett, E. J. (2015). Social support from church and family members and depressive symptoms among older African Americans. *The American Journal of Geriatric Psychiatry, 23*(6), 559–567. https://doi.org/10.1016/j.jagp.2014.04.008

Creswell, J. W., & Creswell, J. D. (2018). *Research design: Qualitative, quantitative, and mixed methods approaches*. Sage.

Enriquez, V. G. (1992). From colonial to liberation psychology: The Philippine experience. Quezon City: University of the Philippines Press.

Fadul, N., Elsayem, A. F., & Bruera, E. (2020). Integration of palliative care into COVID-19 pandemic planning. *BMJ Supportive & Palliative Care, 11*(1), 40–44. https://doi.org/10.1136/bmjspcare-2020-002364

Moustakas, C. (1994). *Phenomenological research methods*. Sage.

Philippine Statistics Authority. (2022). *2022 National Demographic and Health Survey (NDHS)* (PSA Publication series no. PHL_2022_DHS_v01_M). https://microdata.worldbank.org/index.php/catalog/5846#study_desc1684335103457

Segal, J., Robinson, L., & Smith, M. (2023). Coping with grief and loss. *HelpGuide.org*. Retrieved January 29, 2023 from: https://www.helpguide.org/articles/grief/coping-with-grief-and-loss.htm

Sheehan, D. V., Giddens, J. M., & Sheehan, K. H. (2014). Current assessment and classification of suicidal phenomena using the FDA 2012 draft guidance document on suicide assessment: A critical review. *Innovations in Clinical Neuroscience, 11*, 54–65.

Task Force on a Moral Recovery Program (1988, April 27). A Moral Recovery Program: Building a People, Building a Nation. [Submitted to President Corazon Aquino, the Senate, and the members of the press].

Torrens-Burton, A., Goss, S., Sutton, E., Barawi, K., Longo, M., Seddon, K., Carduff, E., Farnell, D. J., Nelson, A., Byrne, A., Phillips, R., Selman, L. E., & Harrop, E. (2022). 'It was brutal. It still is': A qualitative analysis of the challenges of bereavement during the COVID-19 pandemic reported in two national surveys. *Palliative Care and Social Practice, 16*. https://doi.org/10.1177/26323524221092456

van Schaik, P., Leening, H., Stroebe, M., & Schut, H. T. (2022). The effect of the COVID-19 pandemic on grief experiences of bereaved relatives: An overview review. *Research in Social and Administrative Pharmacy, 18*(2), 307–316. https://doi.org/10.1016/j.sapharm.2021.12.011

Walsh, F. (2020). Loss and resilience in the time of COVID-19: Meaning making, hope, and transcendence. *Family Process, 59*(3), 898–911. https://doi.org/10.1111/famp.12588

Weir, K. (2020). *Grief and COVID-19: Saying goodbye in the age of physical distancing*. https://www.apa.org.https://www.apa.org/topics/covid-19/grief-distance

Wong, P. (2017). Death acceptance and the meaning-centered approach to end-of-life care | Dr. Paul Wong. *Drpaulwong.com*. http://www.drpaulwong.com/death-acceptance-meaning-centered-approach-end-life-care/

Yasgur, B. S. (2021, February 17). *A time to grieve: Addressing bereavement challenges during the COVID-19 pandemic*. Psychiatry Advisor. Retrieved June 23, 2022, from https://www.psychiatryadvisor.com/home/topics/generalpsychiatry/a-time-to-grieve-addressing-bereavement-challenges-during-thecovid-19-pandemic/

Zavrou, R., Charalambous, A., Papastavrou, E., Koutrouba, A., & Karanikola, M. (2022). Trying to keep alive a non-traumatizing memory of the deceased: A meta-synthesis on the interpretation of loss in suicide-bereaved family members, their coping strategies and the effects on them. *Journal of Psychiatric and Mental Health Nursing*. https://doi.org/10.1111/jpm.12866

Zhai, Y., & Du, X. (2020). Loss and grief amidst COVID-19: A path to adaptation and resilience. *Brain, Behavior, and Immunity, 87*, 80–81. https://doi.org/10.1016/j.bbi.2020.04.053

# Cabinet of Curiosities: Exploring the Lived Experiences of Selected Filipino Queer Students in-the-Closet

**Gabrielle G Bulahan, Janine Patricia G. Evora, Frances Mikaela A. Llorca, Catherine B. Magno, Raymond Czar C. Mendoza, and Aprilyn E. Calvario**

## Introduction

In the Philippines, the SOGIE bill aims to end gender-based discrimination, but gender is now considered a spectrum rather than a binary. The country's patriarchy, heteronormativity, and patriarchal ideology perpetuate gender roles and expectations, leading to abuse and violence. The LGBT community faces stigma and challenges in schooling due to bullying, discrimination, and lack of access to information. This study explores the experiences of queer college students in-the-closet, aiming to raise awareness among those afraid to express themselves. The study benefits various groups and communities by educating them on how queer individuals live, overcome challenges, and express themselves. The study also adds knowledge to existing studies for future research.

## Methods

This phenomenological study aimed to explore the lived experiences of closed-minded queer college students and their impact on gender expression and identity. The study followed an Interpretative Phenomenological Analysis procedure, analyzing semi-structured interviews and participant descriptions. Emerging themes

G. G. Bulahan · J. P. G. Evora · F. M. A. Llorca · C. B. Magno · R. C. C. Mendoza ·
A. E. Calvario (✉)
Polytechnic University of the Philippines Santa Rosa Laguna Campus,
City of Santa Rosa, Laguna, Philippines
e-mail: ggbulahan@iskolarngbayan.pup.edu.ph; jpgevora@iskolarngbayan.pup.edu.ph;
fmllorca@iskolarngbayan.pup.edu.ph; cbmagno@iskolarngbayan.pup.edu.ph;
rccmendoza@iskolarngbayan.pup.edu.ph; aecalvario@pup.edu.ph

© The Author(s), under exclusive license to Springer Nature Switzerland AG 2024          23
D. Nyaga, R. A. Torres (eds.), *Reimagining Mental Health and Addiction Under the Covid-19 Pandemic,* Volume 1, Advances in Mental Health and Addiction,
https://doi.org/10.1007/978-3-031-58367-4_3

were interpreted using excerpts from interviews to support their justification. The participants of this study focused on students from the Polytechnic University of the Philippines, Santa Rosa Campus (PUP-SRC), a state university in the Philippines, who were enrolled for S.Y. 2022–2023. They were all comfortable discussing their experiences, reasons, challenges, and coping mechanisms related to their gender identity and expressions. The data collected to support the study was done through interviews and audio recordings, while offering options for online conversations, face-to-face conversations in secluded cafes, and classrooms at PUP-SRC. Cameras were not required for privacy. The research instruments were semi-structured questions and underwent face and content validation and were established by consulting three psychology Master's degree holders. During the data gathering procedures, PUP-SRC queer students in-the-closet were informed of the study's nature and objectives and informed of its implications. Participants signed a consent form, which kept interview transcripts private and allowed them to leave the study at any time. Interpretative Phenomenological Analysis (IPA) was utilized to analyze the semi-structured interviews of the study and was validated through a qualitative triangulation method, with a registered psychologist, study participants, and researchers as validators.

## Results and Discussion

### *Definition of in-the-Closet*

Being in-the-closet, as defined by participants, entails differing and varying sets of meanings. Aside from that, those experiences were magnified by the emotions and the thoughts that they had after describing the meaning of their experience. *A reserved gender expression* signifies that when a person is in-the-closet, they have the option to limit what they share to other people, become more cautious, and be reserved in expressing their true gender identity. Living in-the-closet comes with reservation and limitation of one's expression of real behavior, and there is a need to be cautious when interacting with other people. In addition, this phenomenon infers that it is a hindrance toward showing one's true gender identity and expression due to certain reasons, such as fear of being seen and judged based on one's sexuality. Participants view being in-the-closet as a regular occurrence where they select trusted individuals to confide or reveal their authentic gender identity and expression; thus, they can be *selectively out*. Being in-the-closet allows individuals to selectively show their true gender identity to a community they believe they belong to, believing they will be welcomed and not judged. Moreover, being in-the-closet is a *safe space* for individuals to express themselves, especially those who aren't comfortable revealing their gender identity. It offers a safe haven for those who aren't comfortable with expressing their true identity. However, it's not always preferable, as it can also provide protection and a less stressful life. MJ's perception suggests that staying in-the-closet is a convenient way to live a safe life.

## Emerging Reasons for Remaining in-the-Closet

Being in-the-closet results in a reserved expression of the gender identity of the queer students. Thus, they choose to be selectively out only to the people who they consider as their safe space. There is a common theme among all of the participants where they consider themselves as in-the-closet toward certain cohorts: their families and to those who have negative reactions toward queer. Participants from religious families faced judgment and internalized homophobia due to societal expectations rooted from the *instilled religious beliefs of* their family. Participants remained in-the-closet due to conflicting religious and gender identities, causing them to compartmentalize their true gender identity and expression. Furthermore, *patriarchal belief* of the family members has a significant impact on why the participants remain in-the-closet. This can be seen as their family members internally mock queer individuals and lean toward patriarchy—in politics and at home. However, participants still view in-the-closet as a *safe space* due to convenience and security.

## Challenges Experienced in Relation to Being in-the-Closet

The participants faced *religious condemnation* as they grew up in a religiously conservative Filipino community. Fleur, a queer woman, shared her experience of being challenged by her family's religious beliefs and the church's stance on queer people. Kiwi, a religious authority, forbade expressing gender identity that differed from religious norms, highlighting the struggles of holding back one's identity to abide by religious norms. Albert, a queer man, shared his own traumatic experience of holding back his identity. Both participants experienced dissonance between their religious beliefs and accepting their queer identity. In line with this, the participants also faced *family condemnation*, causing difficulties in accepting their gender identity and expression. They also experienced unpleasant comments from family and others. Fleur's experience highlights the struggle to confide in her family about her queer identity, as she felt hurt and hesitant to speak about her true identity. This negative impact on their everyday life highlights the importance of understanding and accepting one's identity. Moreover, the participants experienced *restrictions in social interaction*, feeling cautious and unable to share certain gender information. Socialization is crucial for personal development and emotional health, but without safety, it can limit one's growth. Mj's life challenges involve pretending to be someone they aren't, fearing rejection from family and others. Kiwi, a queer in-the-closet, experienced difficulty coming out and being aware of his surroundings. Because of the gravity of their untold experiences, queer individuals suffered and faced *psychological distress* which resulted in mixed emotions such as intense sadness, anxiety, loneliness, discomfort in social situations, and pain. This had a negative impact on their mental health, which led to significant levels of psychologi-cal distress.

## Influence of Life Challenges to Gender Expression

Given the challenges the participants have had in their lives, it is seen from their experience that they tend to *adapt their gender expression* depending on the circum-stance they were given. The participants faced unique challenges in expressing their gender, with some using writing and self-expression, while others struggle with religious beliefs and trauma. Proactive and reactive gender expressions are influ-enced by life challenges and unique experiences, requiring adaptations to show authentic expression. Consequently, the life challenges influence participants' gen-der expression, often limiting and confining it. They push them to live in *confined gender expression*. Moreover, their convenience with certain people, religious beliefs, trauma, and struggles with societal norms and expectations influences them to have confined gender expression. The participants' responses suggest that the reason they restrict their gender expression is a sense of *safety*. Queer individuals are wary of judgment and discrimination, which can affect their expression. The Philippines' political and sociocultural landscape contributes to the negative stereo-types and negative connotations against the queer community. Despite this, some participants feel safe and inclusive, while others feel unsafe around different groups. Supportive and encouraging individuals can help participants feel safe and important.

## Coping Mechanisms in Relation to the Challenges Experienced

As the queer students experience life challenges in relation to being in-the-closet, they have developed coping mechanisms to deal with them. First, participants often *focus on interests and hobbies*. These coping mechanisms are diverse and can be attributed to various reasons. The participants' reliance on these coping mecha-nisms can be a source of motivation and validation for their personal growth. Secondly, participants in-the-closet as queer students often use *emotional repres-sion* as a coping mechanism, as suppressing emotions can be effective but may be the only option. This limiting behavior may jeopardize their gender identity. Lastly, queer students in-the-closet use *socialization* as a coping mechanism, seeking emo-tional and social support from trusted friends. Their support systems help them communicate feelings, validate their feelings, and maintain a trustworthy personal-ity and sense of security.

# Discussion

## *Definition of in-the-Closet*

Dissociation is a disruption in identity, emotion, perception, body representation, motor control, and behavior. It is often associated with being in-the-closet, where individuals choose to disassociate their identity, body representation, or behavior as a defense mechanism. Castronuevo-Rugas's definition of in-the-closet emphasizes privacy, leading to a sense of hiding a person's gender identity that is nonconforming.

## *Emerging Reasons for Remaining in-the-Closet*

The study by Evangelista et al. (2018) explains the conflict between religious and gender identity among sexual minorities. Participants value their sexual and religious identities, despite their struggles to accept their gender. Despite attempting to constrain their true gender identity through heteronormative behaviors, their religious beliefs continue to manifest and create conflict with their sexual identity. Individuals often face a choice between renouncing their sexuality or relinquishing their religious convictions, leading to internalized homophobia. This self-hatred and guilt are ingrained in the belief system of homosexuals, causing intrapsychic conflict between feelings of needing to be heterosexual and experiences of same-sex attachment or desire. Globally, religiosity has been positively correlated with homophobia, with homophobia and rigid religiosity being strongly associated. Participants faced challenges in accepting their LGBTQ+ community due to patriarchal beliefs and male dominance in their homes. This fear of coming out led to discrimination and fear of being mocked by their family. The issue of sexual orientation and gender identity discrimination also affects politics and social organizations. The LGBT movement has a long history of establishing minority status and attempting to advance its interests in the political sphere. Filipinos are collectivist, prioritizing collective interests over individual ones. They often impose collectivism from family members, requiring them to consider their family's thoughts before revealing their true gender identity. These collectivist countries prioritize the collective's objectives, highlighting the ties that bind members through behaviors and way of life. Marceta (2021) argues that conservative values can limit LGBT people by pressuring them to conform to society's expectations. Students may be motivated to keep their sexual orientation in-the-closet due to their family's traditional values and concern for reactions. Some individuals choose to conceal their sexual minorities to lessen exposure to discrimination and protect themselves from its negative effects.

## Challenges Experienced in Relation to Being in-the-Closet

The Philippines' Christian population has a significant impact on queer Filipinos, leading to homophobic violence and challenges in spirituality and gender identity. Participants are tightly tied to their religious beliefs, resulting in a conscious effort to stray away from their acceptance of their queer identity. The church's opposition to queer people challenges them to remain in-the-closet. Personal construct theory validates these challenges, as they are validated by their traumatic experiences and religious background. Queer individuals have higher rates of adverse religious experiences, leading to religious trauma and negative mental health. Negative views of religion and spirituality can cause unresolvable conflict within the queer community and fractured identity formation. Many queer individuals struggle to reconcile their spiritual and sexual identities, leading to their "closet" status. Steinberg and Duncan (2002) emphasize the importance of positive and familial relationships for youth's well-being. However, many queer youths fear coming out to their parents, leading to family condemnation. This fear can result in unwanted rejection and denial of same-gender attraction. Docena (2013) found that coming out to parents was the most challenging aspect, as individuals suppress same-gender attraction and try to act straight. The fear of parental rejection and the perception of being gay made it difficult for participants to express and share their true identity. ASEAN SOGIE Caucus (2017) highlights the prevalence of rejection and psychological trauma for queers, often originating from family and relatives. This theme is linked to the personal construct theory, where individuals prioritize their family and personal constructs, leading to difficulties with family relationships and a lack of acceptance. Ereno's study found that participants who selectively disclose their gender identity struggle with self-discovery in a culture that treats homosexuals as outcasts. This leads to issues like low self-esteem, depression, and social avoidance. Queer teens experience more depressive symptoms than heterosexual teens, with factors like vulnerability, nonconformity, family rejection, and homophobia contributing to distress. Internalized stigma, fear of disclosure, and identity concealment can also contribute to these issues. Factors like closetedness, family rejection, and homophobia contribute to the distress experienced by queer youth.

## Influence of Life Challenges to Gender Expression

Based on the preceding statements, the theory of gender performativity by Judith Butler (1999) supports the following inferences. As mentioned, gender performativity claims that gender and gender roles are elaborate social performances that people present to certain individuals depending on the social context. The experiences of queer students in-the-closet reflect this theory in a way that their elaborate social performance comes into play in a form of adaptive gender expression. As brought by their life challenges, their gender becomes a performance whenever they feel like they have to adapt to certain situations, factors, or stimuli by modifying their expression of their gender identity. Lee's study reveals that coping mechanisms, such as self-control and denial defenses, are used to conceal actions and behavior. These psychological mechanisms contribute to the confinement of gender expression in the closet, allowing participants to avoid judgment from family, friends, and society. Coleman highlighted discrimination against the LGBTQ community in 201,954, stating that majority culture is hostile toward LGBTQ individuals. This prejudice disrupts their well-being and causes them to face unfavorable adversities. LGBTQ students are more likely to experience violence and poor health due to negative views. Coleman concluded that laws and policies are necessary for LGBTQ equality but insufficient. Transgender people often conceal their gender expressions due to fear of adverse reactions, assault, or prejudice. Internal conflict makes anxiety, sadness, suicide, and self-harm more likely.

## Coping Mechanisms in Relation to the Challenges Experienced

This emerging theme is connected to the study of Hazel et al. (2022). Self-determination theory and flow state are psychological mechanisms that help players cope with their emotions and experiences in online games. Autonomy involves controlling the avatar's actions and personality, while competence involves dealing with frustration and overcoming obstacles. Relatedness involves connecting with other players or in-game characters, while flow is a state where people are so engrossed in a task that nothing else seems important. These mechanisms contribute to positive affect, enhanced performance, reduced anxiety, and elevated self-esteem. Studies have shown that students cope with their LGBTQ identities by focusing on academics and using their skills in writing, music, and leadership. Emotion-focused coping, such as positive self-talk, positive reconceptualization of stressful events, altering negative thoughts, and acceptance, can help gay men manage their internal emotional state. Garcia's (2012) study emphasizes concealing gender orientation, which involves hiding one's sexual orientation to avoid revealing their identity. Situation modification coping, such as concealing one's sexual orientation and maintaining a hidden profile in a heterosexist environment, is employed when the source of stress cannot be changed. In-the-closet coping mechanisms involve suppressing emotions and distance, with self-control and distancing being the main coping strategies. These mechanisms help participants manage their emotions and maintain a sense of belonging in online games. The study by Hutcheson (2012) highlights the importance of a support system consisting of friends, family, teachers, and gay-straight alliances. Positive coping, such as participation in peer support groups, is linked to the emerging theme. Emotion-focused coping involves emotional disclosure, seeking social support, and acceptance, enabling gay men to manage their internal emotional state.

# Conclusion

The way the Filipino queer students in-the-closet define the term in-the-closet entails double-edged meanings as their notion toward this concept includes both positive and negative connotations. Their definitions were rooted from their perceived experiences as someone who is in-the-closet. Based on the perceived experiences of Filipino queer students in-the-closet, the common denominator on the reasons why they remain in-the-closet is due to the societal expectations from their social environment that penetrate deep within their gender identity and gender expression. Also, they encounter external challenges in their daily lives which cost internal psychological conflicts. Furthermore, the life challenges experienced by the Filipino queer students in-the-closet influenced their gender expression by adapting, confining, and shifting gender expression in the form of psychological defense mechanisms such as dissociation, self-control, and denial defenses. They shift their gender expression by depending their behavior on certain factors such as the person(s) they are with, the safety they will feel, and the place or the environment they are situated with at a given time. Lastly, Filipino queer students in-the-closet cope with life's challenges in relation to being in-the-closet through negative and positive coping mechanisms. They coped through focusing on interests, emotional repression, and socialization.

The researchers of this study recommend that the queer youth are encouraged to join seminars, forums, and discussions that talk about their struggles and challenges, to have an outlet in the form of journaling or by joining social group forums or focus group discussion. Families and friends are encouraged to actively engage in conversation and discussion, to read and research studies about queer in-the-closet and to attend gender sensitivity programs or training and also express displeasure toward slurs or jokes based on gender, gender identity, or sexual orientation, whether it may be in the community or media. Schools and communities must integrate topics such as gender sensitivity training courses in NSTP programs, create safe spaces for queer youth, and implement guidance counselors that may develop programs related to their challenges and needs. Government institutions and barangay local government units are encouraged to make better reinforcement of existing policies pertaining to queer safe spaces. Barangay level may reconsider having dialogue with school authorities and officials about the implementation of House Bill No. 5562. Future researchers must conduct additional investigation and revision of this study by exploring more on the connection of gender expression toward their sexual orientation, use other demographics aside from students as participants, and utilize a longitudinal study.

# References

ASEAN SOGIE Caucus. (2017). *The rainbow in context: An overview of the situation of lesbian, gay, bisexual, transgender, intersex, and queer (LGBTIQ) persons in Southeast Asia*. Retrieved from: https://aseansogiecaucus.org/images/2017/ASC_Rainbow_in_Context_LGBTIQ_Persons_in_SEA.pdf

Butler, J. (1999). *Gender trouble: Feminism and the subversion of identity* (Rev ed.). Routledge.

Docena, P. (2013). *Developing and managing one's sexual identity: Coming out stories of Waray Gay adolescents*. Retrieved from: https://www.academia.edu/27447495/Developing_and_Managing_Ones_Sexual_Identity_Coming_Out_Stories_of_Waray_Gay_Adolescents

Evangelista, Z. M., Dumaop, D. E., & Nelson, G. (2018). *Journeying to a safe space: Sexual and religious identity integration of Filipino LGBT-affirmative church members*. www.semanticscholar.org. Retrieved from: https://www.semanticscholar.org/paper/Journeying-to-a-Safe-Space-%3A-Sexual-and-Religious-Evangelisa-Dumaop/44b81778bfcf668c3dc2baf76918168fe04995a7

Garcia, H. B. (2012). *Supporting lesbian, gay, and bisexual youth in high school: A retrospective study*. Saint Mary's College of California ProQuest Dissertations Publishing, 2012.1514527. Retrieved from: https://www.proquest.com/openview/e72aadce1811d639b716b91a1c0baf95/1?pq-origsite=gscholar&cbl=18750

Hazel, J., Kim, H. M., & Every-Palmer, S. (2022). Exploring the possible mental health and wellbeing benefits of video games for adult players: A cross-sectional study. *Australasian Psychiatry, 30*(4), 541–546. https://journals.sagepub.com/doi/pdf/10.1177/10398562221103081

Hutcheson, V. H. (2012). *Dealing with dual differences: Social coping strategies of gifted and lesbian, gay, bisexual, transgender, and queer adolescents*. Dissertations, theses, and masters projects. Paper 1539272210. https://doi.org/10.25774/w4-bwnw-qg16

Marceta, J. (2021). *Individualism under constraining social norms: Conceptualizing the lived experiences of LGBT persons*. Retrieved from: https://philarchive.org/archive/MARIUC

Steinberg, L., & Duncan, P. (2002). Work group IV: Increasing the capacity of parents, families, and adults living with adolescents to improve adolescent health outcomes. *The Journal of Adolescent Health, 31*, 261–263.

# Breathe Out: Ecopsychology and Eco-anxiety Relating to Age, Sex, and Climate Crisis Knowledge

**April Mae O. Evangelista, Shaira Mae A. David, Jill B. Diaz, Marinard C. Florendo, Kristel Joy B. Triveles, Aprilyn E. Calvario, and Donnies Bendicio**

## Introduction

The uprising of online and physical climate protests worldwide was due to an eye-opening event that happened on April 6 of the same year, when a NASA scientist and three other scientists were arrested after chaining themselves to the doors of a Chase Bank office building in Los Angeles (McFall-Johnsen, 2022). Peter Kalmus, a climate scientist at NASA, fought off his tears in a video of his speech that warned everyone on the planet about the impending destruction of the Earth in less than 5 years.

> This is for all of the kids of the world, all of the young people, all of the future people.

> The world only has less than five years before it ends.

These sentences, said by NASA scientists, inflicted fear on people, especially those who spend a lot of time on the Internet. Most believed that they were too young to have the world end after 5 years. They experienced worry, fear, powerlessness, and anxiety in that instant realization that the world is, in fact, dying. Climate change has an effect on people's emotions and perceptions. Findings indicate that emotions need to be specifically related to the climate problem to have significant behavioral effects (Brosch, 2021). The more people care about their lives, the higher the

A. M. O. Evangelista · S. M. A. David · J. B. Diaz · M. C. Florendo · K. J. B. Triveles
A. E. Calvario (✉)
Polytechnic University of the Philippines Santa Rosa Laguna Campus, City of Santa Rosa, Laguna, Philippines
e-mail: amoevangelista@iskolarngbayan.pup.edu.ph; smadavid@iskolarngbayan.pup.edu.ph; jbdiaz@iskolarngbayan.pup.edu.ph; mcflorendo@iskolarngbayan.pup.edu.ph; kjbtriveles@iskolarngbayan.pup.edu.ph; aecalvario@pup.edu.ph

D. Bendicio
Lahok Training Center, Bacoor, Philippines

© The Author(s), under exclusive license to Springer Nature Switzerland AG 2024
D. Nyaga, R. A. Torres (eds.), *Reimagining Mental Health and Addiction Under the Covid-19 Pandemic,* Volume 1, Advances in Mental Health and Addiction,
https://doi.org/10.1007/978-3-031-58367-4_4

chances are that they will worry about the future of the world. According to Agnew (2022), the worry that people feel about the planet's status today is not just about the status itself but also the lack of response to it. It is stated that the more we understand the situation, the more we worry about the future and its bad effects in the upcoming years. The Society for Environmental, Population, and Conservation Psychology, also called APA Division 34, stated that issues related to climate change have significant mental health impacts. The worry, fear, anxiety, and hopelessness about the impacts of the deteriorating health of the Earth, either constantly or temporarily, is called "eco-anxiety" (Adutt, 2020). The American Psychological Association defined eco-anxiety as "the chronic fear of environmental cataclysm that comes from observing the seemingly irrevocable impact of climate change and the associated concern for one's future and that of next generations," in which they considered the different environmental problems that can lead to psychological consequences that vary in seriousness in a wide range of people (Iberdrola, 2022). Although the term "eco-anxiety" has not been classified in the DSM-5, it has been used in academic textbooks and media since 2007 but not until 2016 when an increasing need for eco-therapy arose as people talked in their therapy sessions about being indecisive on life-changing decisions, specifically having children in the future because of the quality of life (Whitcomb, 2021). A survey conducted in the United States reported that over 45% of 10,000 16- to 25-year-olds in 10 countries said that their feelings about climate change negatively affected their daily lives and functioning (Whiting, 2021). In 2020, the American Psychiatric Association posted a poll that revealed that 67% of Americans were extremely anxious about the impacts of climate change, and more than half of them were extremely anxious about its effect on their mental health. The United Kingdom's RC Psych (2020) found out that 57% of child and adolescent psychiatrists were seeing children and young people being distressed about the climate crisis and the planet's status.

This study is based on Dodds' (2021) one of the four psychological hypotheses for why people do not act against one of the biggest threats that the world is facing these days—the climate crisis, which is the disconnection of human beings from nature. But through the recent developments in the digital era that the world is in now, the connection to nature has been strengthened by people's mobilization and virtual protests about different environmental issues that the world is currently facing. Ecopsychologists emphasized that our anxiousness, remorse, despair, and frustration about the destruction of ecosystems and the pain for the planet are all valid, and they provide the starting point for action and a renewed relationship with the Earth. Thus, reconnecting to nature is seen as a requirement for mental health that also provides the emotional link that will drive us to act. With this theory, the researchers will tackle the connections between participants' age, sex, and knowledge about the climate crisis in ecopsychology. Psychoanalyst Harold Searles (1972) suggested that "a human is hampered in his meeting of this environmental crisis by a severe and pervasive apathy, which is based upon feelings and attitudes of which he is unconscious." Pihkala (2018) described eco-anxiety as "various difficult emotions and mental states arising from environmental conditions and knowledge about them." With the lack of studies or research in the field of this certain phenomenon, Pihkala used the term "environmental anxiety." "Worry and anxiety" are technically distinct mental states, but they are inextricably linked when it comes to climate change and other environmental issues. With this theory, the researchers will tackle the connections between participants' age, sex, and their level of knowledge about the climate crisis in a country that is known to be the most disaster-prone place to be in the middle of the climate crisis effects.

The study was intended to conduct additional research about ecopsychology and eco-anxiety in the Philippines, specifically in Region IV-A, the most populous region in the country, which was far less researched in a place that is prone to the effects of climate change. Its purpose was to determine the ecopsychology and the eco-anxiety relationships with the residents of Region IV-A regarding their age, sex, and knowledge about the climate crisis. The study solely focuses on the relationships of both ecopsychology and eco-anxiety to age, sex, and climate crisis knowledge of the CALABARZON residents. Respondents to the research will be Filipinos who currently live in CALABARZON. Filipinos who are currently abroad aren't allowed to take part in the study. The study benefits the Filipino people, as most of them are not aware of ecopsychology and eco-anxiety. This research would help the government identify knowledge gaps among citizens regarding the climate crisis, thereby improving sustainable environmental goals and increasing climate crisis awareness. It can help them with mental health preparations in times of a climate crisis and/or disasters influenced by climate change. On a specific note, for the Department of Education and Commission on Higher Education, this study can also serve as instructional reading material about ecopsychology, eco-anxiety, and the climate crisis that can help the institution promote awareness of the environment and the current crisis that threatens the Philippines. The item difficulty available in the analysis of this study can provide a glimpse of what can be added to the learning materials of the current subjects implemented in the country. The information gathered and the results in this study can lead to future new topics and areas, such as getting more specific into the demographic profile of the respondents, educational attainment, the provinces or municipalities, and grassroots level, the age groups like elementary, high school, and college, which are based on the educational system in the country, that future researchers can cover related to the climate crisis, eco-anxiety, and ecopsychology in the Philippines and the rest of the world.

## Experimental Method/s

In conducting the study, the researchers used a quantitative (correlational) research design to determine the relationship of eco-anxiety and ecopsychology in relation to age, sex, and knowledge about the climate crisis of the participants. The participants are Filipinos residing in Region IV-A, belonging to the age group of adolescents (10–19 years old) and adults (above 19 years old). A probability sampling technique was used, specifically the simple random sampling technique. Participants filled out a Google Form online that accumulated 302 participants, and with the use of

G*Power, a sample size of 138 was determined. To get the 138 respondents out of the 302 population, the 302 participants were assigned a number chronologically, and then 138 respondents were randomly drawn from the 302 population. The research instrument consisted of the Climate Change Anxiety Scale (Clayton & Karazsia, 2020), the Connectedness to Nature Scale (Mayer & McPherson Frantz, 2005), and the Climate Change Knowledge Assessment (EARTHDAY.ORG, 2021), which was used after asking permission from the authors and having qualified validators validate the questionnaire. To gather the data needed, the research instrument was disseminated online with the use of a Google Form. After collecting and compiling the data, the chi-square rest for independence, item difficulty, mean, and weighted mean were used to analyze it.

## Results and Discussion

**Profile of the Participants** The knowledge level of the participants. More than half of the respondents have low-level knowledge about the climate crisis, with most of them scoring 7 out of 11 on the Climate Change Knowledge Scale. The education system in the Philippines established climate competencies integrated with cocurricular activities across grade levels (DepEd, 2020), but despite these, the results presented above agree with the study of Bolletino et al. (2020), which states that Filipinos have low levels of knowledge about the climate crisis, whereas 62.1% of their respondents from Region IV-A "haven't heard nor are well-informed" about the matter at hand. Adults have a higher knowledge level than adolescents. In a narrative synthesized by Lee et al. (2019) on youth's perception of climate change, the results above give evidence to the previous study's reports, which stated that the younger the age, the less accurate their knowledge is about the climate crisis. The results also aligned with a study from Southeast Asia conducted by Sulistyawati et al. (2017), which provided a shred of evidence that there's a "low and inconsistent understanding" regarding climate change in adolescents. Also, females have higher knowledge level than males. In an explainer published by UN Women (2022), the climate crisis is stated to be "not gender neutral" since women experience climate change's greatest impacts. Almost half of the Philippine delegates to the Conference of Parties event annually consisted of women, describing them as "key agents of change"; hence, women's participation in decision-making processes at local and national levels is indispensable (Philippine Commission on Women, 2020). The result also agrees with the study on population and environment by McCright (2010), which revealed women convey greater scientific knowledge about climate change compared to men.

**Items Difficult for the Respondents to Answer** UNESCO (2022) emphasizes that to promote climate action, education about the climate crisis and its impacts is crucial. Although the Philippines has been implementing climate competencies in the country's education system and also boosting the dissemination of information through an additional subject in senior high school, with the analysis of item difficulty results, the study provides information on what educators should focus on more—the statistics of climate crisis impacts than the non-changeable knowledge.

**Level of Eco-anxiety of the Respondents**   From the most recent studies involving respondents from the Philippines in eco-anxiety, also known as climate anxiety, climate distress in the respondents is evident (Hickman, 2021), like how the eco-anxiety data is tabulated above. Looking back at the geographic region of the Philippines, most Filipinos have experienced disastrous typhoons that impact the livelihood of most individuals, especially their homes. In the CALABARZON region, most of the houses are either near or beside the mountain or house built beside the river or lake, thus most of the residents nearby experienced flash floods, landslides, etc. that even took the lives of the individuals. Based on the analysis of the data treated, adults have a greater average rate than adolescents but with the same minimum and maximum levels of eco-anxiety. Given that everyone is dependent on the planet's health, eco-anxiety may impact anybody, but it does not affect everyone in the same way. As a result, some people may have increased concern about climate change. According to the World Health Organization (2021), certain populations suffer a higher risk of eco-anxiety because they are more vulnerable to climate change. Along with those vulnerable and at risk are adults. Results indicate that females have a greater mean than males; thus the result shows different climate change anxiety between the sexes of the respondents. A research mapping published in Carbon Brief by Dunne (2020) from 130 studies around the world suggested that women are more susceptible to climate-driven mental disorders since they are the most affected sector when it comes to the effects of the climate crisis. Three studies in the local setting provided evidence that females are the ones who are most likely to suffer following the effects of climate change in the Philippines. Morrow (2014) found poor reproductive and maternal health after being exposed to typhoons. Food insecurity (Anttila-Hughes & Hsiang, 2013) has affected females in terms of mortality more than males because of the scarcity of food in families; Ballera et al. (2015) studied the demographics during Super Typhoon Haiyan and made the discovery that women are 50% more likely to die or be injured from extreme weather in the country. The high-level knowledge has a greater mean than low-level knowledge, and thus the result gives a different level of climate change anxiety between the knowledge levels of the respondents. This implies that most citizens who are unaware of the climate crisis have low levels of eco-anxiety. The Harvard Humanitarian Initiative (HHI) discovered that Filipinos had a low degree of public knowledge regarding climate change. Most respondents (60% on average) had not heard of it and did not feel well-informed about it, while just 12% had heard a lot about it or felt "very well-informed" about it. According to the survey, Filipinos who view climate change as having a direct influence on their homes take more precautions to prepare for disasters. Filipinos who think they have been personally influenced by climate-related changes are more inclined to prepare for disasters, make plans, and take certain precautions, such as home modifications. Anyone who has access to information about climate change via modern communications technology may be at risk of developing this anxiety reaction (Reyes et al., 2021). The mean and standard deviation on the eco-anxiety level felt by the respondents and the result indicate that the highest rank was "My friends say I do not think about climate change too much." with a mean and standard deviation of (WM = 3.51, SD = 1.29), which was being interpreted by the respondents as "often," and the last rank was "I write down my thoughts about climate change and analyze them" with a mean and standard deviation of (WM = 1.96, SD = 1.15), which was being interpreted as "rarely." The overall mean was 2.75 and had a standard deviation of 1.21; it was being interpreted as "sometimes." Feather and Williams (2022) measured the psychometric properties of the CCAS and mentioned that Clayton and Karazsia produced a 13-item scale to measure eco-anxiety, whereas items 1–8 are for cognitive-emotional impairment, while items 9–13 are for functional impairment factors. Based on the responses gathered and presented above, most of the participants are not eliciting both cognitive-emotional and functional impairments.

**Level of Ecopsychology of the Respondents** The distribution of participants' ecopsychology levels is presented. 63 of 138 CALABARZON residents have been connected to nature based on the CNS rating and interpretation; most of the participants are connected to nature. Only 23.19% of the sample was sometimes connected to nature or sometimes disconnected from it. A previous study has shown that individuals' exposure to, or connection with, nature can influence their levels of connectedness to the environment (Anderson & Krettenauer, 2021). Several explanations have been presented to explain why time spent in nature and emotional attachment to the environment are connected. The ecopsychology of the respondents according to age group and the result indicate that adolescents have a mean and standard deviation of (WM = 3.03, SD = 0.78), while adults have a mean and standard deviation of WM = 3.30, SD = 0.74, which was interpreted as "sometimes connected to nature, sometimes disconnected from nature" with a minimum level of 1.86 and a maximum level of 4.43. The result indicates that adults have a greater mean than adolescents; thus, the result gives a different ecopsychology between the age groups of the respondents. According to a study conducted by Anderson and Krettenauer (2021), individuals who spent time in nature frequently as children were shown to be more likely to engage in pro-environmental behavior than those who did not. The effect of age, sex, and the living situation on emotional connectedness to nature and pro-environmental behavior was investigated in this research. Contrary to the research's results, adolescents and adults have a similar level of connectedness to nature. It was revealed that the ecopsychology of the respondents according to sex and the result indicate that females have a mean and standard deviation of (WM = 3.46, SD =0.58), which is being interpreted as "connected to nature" with a minimum level of 1.93 and a maximum level of 4.43. Adults have a mean and standard deviation of (WM = 2.95, SD =0.83), which is interpreted as "sometimes connected to nature, Sometimes Disconnected from Nature," with a minimum level of 1.86 and a maximum level of 4.50. The result indicates that females have a greater mean than males, thus indicating a different ecopsychology between the sexes of the respondents. Men are less concerned about the environment than women because of the presence of dominance not just in the workplace but also in fighting the climate crisis, as cited by Pease (2019) in their study which focuses on being more concerned about environmentalism. Scannell and Gifford (2013) also cited in their study that being female is associated with higher personal issues, attitudes, and behaviors. Capaldi et al. (2014) proved this wrong by conducting a meta-analysis and concluded that being female does not give the same results despite the previous research. Meanwhile, Nisbet (2021) found out that sex was relevant to any sense of well-being or connectedness to nature. According to Desrochers et al. (2019), females were more conscientious (i.e., goal-directed and organized) than males. Based on these personality characteristics, females were more likely to promote environmental protection and less likely to support environmental utilization. Conscientiousness also explained why females were more likely than males to participate in pro-environmental behaviors. When masculine and feminine qualities were compared, more feminine individuals were more conscientious and more inclined to participate in pro-environmental activities. The data also shows that the ecopsychology of the respondents according to their knowledge level and the result indicate that high-level knowledge has a mean and standard deviation of (WM = 3.65, SD =0.56), which is being interpreted as "connected to nature" with a minimum level of 1.86 and a maximum level of 4.50. Low-level knowledge has a mean and standard deviation of (WM = 2.80, SD =0.70), which was interpreted as "sometimes connected to nature, sometimes disconnected from nature" with a minimum level of 1.86 and a maximum level of 4.36. The result indicates that high-level knowledge has a greater average mean than low-level knowledge, and thus the result gives a different ecopsychology between the knowledge levels of the respondents. Pereira et al. (2015) state that lack of knowledge is the reason why people act less in an environmentally friendly way, as cited in previous studies that align with the results above. The mean and standard deviation on ecopsychology and the result indicate that the highest rank was "I recognize and appreciate the intelligence of other living organisms." with a mean and standard deviation of (WM = 3.67, SD = 1.07), which was interpreted by the respondents as "agree," and the last rank was "My personal welfare is independent of the welfare of the natural world." with a mean and standard deviation of (WM = 2.69, SD = 1.36), which was being interpreted as "neutral." The overall mean was 3.21 with a standard deviation of 1.16 and was being interpreted as "neutral." Mayer and McPherson Frantz (2005) subjected their developed Connectedness to Nature Scale to five validity and reliability tests, which supported the contention that being connected to nature predicts ecological behavior and the subjective well-being of a person. Based on the given analysis of the responses to the scale, it shows that most participants acknowledge their environment by appreciating the intelligence of other organisms and they believe that their well-being is dependent on the status of the nature or environment they lived in.

**Relationship Between Eco-anxiety to Age, Sex, and Knowledge About the Climate Crisis** The analysis showed the relationship of eco-anxiety felt by the respondents to age group, sex, and knowledge about the climate crisis, and the result indicates that the eco-anxiety level of the respondents has a significant relationship to the sex of the respondents with chi-square value and significance of ($\chi^2$ = 64.867, $p$ = 0.008), respectively, which was being interpreted as significant for the significance or p-value computed which is less than 0.05 level of significance. According to the World Health Organization (2014) and Intergovernmental Panel on Climate Change, women are prone to vulnerability to climate change impact due to their perceived relative lack of power when facing a threat in many cultures. Likewise, women suffer more anxiety and stress than men presumably owing to hormonal factors, evolutionary influences, or gender-specific trauma. There have been reports of women being more concerned and distressed than men in response to climate change. It was also found in a poll conducted by YouGov among Britons concerning the implication of climate change that the biggest difference in levels of eco-anxiety was seen between men and women rather than between rich and poor or young and old. 45% of female participants expressed high levels of worry about climate change compared to 36% of men (Helm, 2021). Likewise, according to Roberts and Lauchlan (2020) research on exploring consumer eco-anxiety and environmental behaviors, 71% of women indicated that thinking about the environment made them nervous, compared to 63% of men. 56% of women felt guilty about their effect on the environment, compared to 45% of men. Women have traditionally been nurturing and caring for their families and have always been concerned with issues of life and death. They have greater tendencies for prosocial, altruistic, and empathetic behaviors that cause them to be concerned about environmental issues and be vulnerable to nature being destroyed (Hunt, 2020). According to the Pew Research Center's Global Attitudes Spring 2015 survey among 11 developing countries around the world, women are more likely to be concerned that global climate change will harm them. There's a difference between knowing and feeling climate change; women feel the danger that we're in emotionally and psychologically (Bury, 2022). Women have more significant stress and anxiety as they are more behaviorally engaged with higher rates of post-traumatic stress disorder (PTSD) following a disaster compared to men. Meanwhile, the chi-square value and significance of ($\chi^2$ = 44.523, $p$ = 0.287) age and eco-anxiety have no significant relationship. According to Roberts and Lauchlan (2020), age was a less obvious predictor of eco-anxiety. Worries about the environment scores across all age groups were high—44% of Gen X (born 1965–1979), 55% of Millennials (born 1980–1995), and 55% of Gen Z (born 1996–2010). The results showed a significant relationship to the knowledge level of the respondents with a chi-square value and significance of ($\chi^2$ = 60.286, $p$ = 0.021). Individuals who know about climate change and its effects can elicit a wide range of emotions, including guilt, sadness, and anger, all of which contribute to eco-anxiety (Pihkala, 2020b). Certain experiences, knowledge, and types of exposure appear to cause eco-anxiety. Naturalists and climate scientists, for example, suffer from eco-anxiety as a result of their knowledge and emotional attachments to the natural world. Fritze et al. (2008) stated that exposure to climate change information regularly such as through social media leads to higher rates of eco-anxiety. Knowing the consequences of climate change can be so worrying that people react with skepticism and denial.

**Relationship Between Ecopsychology to Age, Sex, and Knowledge About the Climate Crisis**   The analysis reveals the significant relationship of ecopsychology to age group, sex, and knowledge about the climate crisis, and the result indicates that ecopsychology has a significant relationship to the sex and knowledge level of the respondents with chi-square values and significance of ($\chi^2 = 63.667$, $p = 0.003$) and ($\chi^2 = 69.136$, $p = 0.001$), respectively, which were interpreted as significant for the significance or p-value computed which is less than 0.05 level of significance. Ecopsychology and age group showed that there is no significant relationship between the two. While both sex and knowledge about the climate crisis showed a significant relationship to ecopsychology, both age groups, adolescents and adults, did not show any significant relationship to ecopsychology. According to the study of Metsäranta (2021), age and eco-anxiety have a slight negative relationship, which suggests that as a person grows older, the eco-anxiety drops, while sex and ecopsychology have a significant relationship, showing that females are more connected to nature compared to males, which showed that males are sometimes connected to nature and sometimes not. Furthermore, the World Health Organization (2014) stated that women are more vulnerable to the effects of climate change than men. Women suffer from anxiety and stress more than men, due to hormonal factors, evolutionary influences, or gender-specific trauma. Females are also found to have more positive views toward developing solutions to environmental issues such as climate change compared to males (Tranter & Skrbis, 2011; Torgleret al., 2008; Uitto et al., 2004; Yilmaz et al., 2004). Similar to sex, knowledge about the climate crisis also showed a significant relationship to ecopsychology. According to Metsäranta (2021), higher education was associated with people being more conscious of climate change issues. The study done by Bolletino (2020) showed that 71% of Filipinos feel that climate change will affect them at least "slightly." Filipinos are also found to have a low level of public awareness about climate change. Despite this statement from the study, Filipinos are very much aware of how climate change may affect them.

## Conclusion

Residents in Region IV-A have inadequate knowledge of the climate crisis, with varying levels of knowledge among age and gender groups. Females are more anxious about climate change effects, while highly informed individuals worry more about the environment. There is a moderate level of connection to nature among residents, with females being more connected than males. Increased knowledge of the climate crisis leads to higher levels of eco-anxiety and connection to nature. Therefore, it is recommended that Filipinos learn more about the climate crisis, the government should invest in environmental projects and policies, and the education system incorporate updated climate facts into curricula. Future research should focus on investigating the relationship between eco-anxiety and ecopsychology and profiling other demographic groups. Additionally, tests and scales should be developed locally to measure eco-anxiety and ecopsychology among Filipinos.

**Acknowledgments** This study is the product of the researchers' hard work and efforts. The researchers want to express their sincere gratitude and appreciation to everyone who has supported and helped them along the way to make this study possible:

The Almighty God, for giving them strength, energy, and the hope that they will finish their study.
To the parents of the researchers, for continuously giving their support and words of encouragement that made the research possible.
To their friends and classmates, for the wonderful experience.
To the respondents, for their time and cooperation in taking part in the study.
To Mr. Donnies Bendicio, for the guidance, support, and sharing of your knowledge, expertise, and insight into the study as the research adviser.
To the faculty for giving words of encouragement for the research to be able to finish the study.
To their statistician, for endless support and insights regarding the statistical treatment and computation of the data as the researchers' statistician.
To Asst Prof Aprilyn Calvario, for the wonderful insight as the Research Professor.
To the panelists for sharing their expertise during the research defense.

# References

Adutt, S. (2020). What is eco-anxiety? *Eco-Anxiety.* https://www.ecoanxiety.com/whatis-eco-anxiety/

Agnew, M. (2022). Welcome to the age of eco-anxiety. *ELLE.* https://www.elle.com/uk/life-and-culture/a39490079/eco-anxiety-mental-health/#

Anderson, D. J., & Krettenauer, T. (2021). Connectedness to nature and pro-environmental behaviour from early adolescence to adulthood: A comparison of urban and rural Canada. MDPI. https://doi.org/10.3390/su13073655

Anttila-Hughes, J., & Hsiang, S. (2013). Destruction, disinvestment, and death: Economic and human losses following environmental disaster. Social Science Research Network. https://doi.org/10.2139/ssrn.2220501

Ballera, J. E., et al. (2015). Management of the dead in Tacloban City after Typhoon Haiyan. *Western Pacific Surveillance and Response, 6*(5). https://doi.org/10.5365/wpsar.2015.6.2.HYN_004

Bolletino, V., et al. (2020). Public perception of climate change and disaster preparedness: Evidence from The Philippines. Elsevier. https://doi.org/10.1016/j.crm.2020.100250

Brosch, T. (2021). Affect and emotions as drivers of climate change perception and action: A review. Science Direct. https://doi.org/10.1016/j.cobeha.2021.02.001

Clayton, S., & Karazsia, B. T. (2020). Psychological Aspects of Environmental Issues.

Co, M., et al. (2014). *Impact assessment of climate change in Quezon Province (Real-Infanta-General Nakar)* (p. 4). Environmental and Climate Change Research Institute, University Research Center, De La Salle Araneta University. https://www.dlsu.edu.ph/wp-content/uploads/pdf/conferences/research-congress-proceedings/2014/SEE/SEE-III-024-FT.pdf

Department of Education. (2020). *The need for climate change education*. GOVPH. https://www.deped.gov.ph/climate-change-education/cce-in-the-philippines/

Desrochers, J., et al. (2019). Does personality mediate the relationship between sex and environmentalism? *Personality and Individual Differences, 147*. https://www.wgtn.ac.nz/__data/assets/pdf_file/0011/1776422/Why_do_women_care_more_about_the_environment_than_men.pdf#:~:text=In%20all%20three%20studies%2C%20females%20were%20more%20conscientious,traits%20also%20showed%20the%20same%20result%20%E2%80%94%20those

Dodds, J. (2021). *The psychology of climate anxiety*. National Library of Medicine: National Center for Biotechnology Information. https://www.ncbi.nlm.nih.gov/pmc/articles/PMC8499625/

Dunne, D. (2020). Mapped: How climate change disproportionately affects women's health. *Carbon Brief Clear on Climate Features*. https://www.carbonbrief.org/mapped-how-climate-change-disproportionately-affects-womens-health/

EARTHDAY.ORG. (2021). The Earthday Official Site. https://www.earthday.org/?ad_source-=1&gclid=CjwKCAjwjqWzBhAqEiwAQmtgT2MIoSK71Qy8asPQ7iaKqBLdfZuORFfVldbtCXby7fM2Ds0EREY7MRoCN7gQAvD_BwE.

Feather, G. & Williams, M. N. (2022). A psychometric evaluation of the Climate Change Anxiety Scale. *PsyArXiv* Preprints. https://doi.org/10.31234/osf.io/uzf7j

Helm, T. (2021). Eco-anxiety over climate crisis suffered by all ages and classes. *The Guardian*. https://www.theguardian.com/environment/2021/oct/31/eco-anxiety-over-climate-crisis-suffered-by-all-ages-and-classes

Hickman, C. (2021). Climate anxiety in children and young people and their beliefs about government responses to climate change: A global survey. *The Lancet Planetary Health*. https://doi.org/10.1016/S2542-5196(21)00278-3

Iberdrola. (2022). *Eco-ansiedade: as sequelas psicológicas da crise climática*. Iberdrola. https://www.iberdrola.com/socialecoanxiety#:%7E:text=The%20American%20Psychology%20Association%20

Lee, K., et al. (2019). Youth perceptions of climate change: A narrative synthesis. *Wiley Interdisciplinary Reviews*. https://doi.org/10.1002/wcc.641

Mayer, S., & McPherson Frantz, C. (2005). The connectedness to nature scale: A measure of individuals' feeling in community with nature. Elsevier. https://www.researchgate.net/profile/Cynthia-Frantz/publication/222621038_The_Connectedness_to_Nature_Scale_A_Measure_of_Individuals'_Feeling_in_Community_with_Nature/links/59fb3664458515d0706069ea/The-Connectedness-to-Nature-Scale-A-Measure-of-Individuals-Feeling-in-Community-with-Nature.pdf?_sg%5B0%5D=started_experiment_milestone&origin=journal

McCright, A. M. (2010). The effects of gender on climate change knowledge and concern in the American public. *Population and Environment, 32*, 66–87. https://doi.org/10.1007/s11111-010-0113-1

McFall-Johnsen, M. (2022). NASA scientist arrested after chaining himself to Chase Bank as part of global climate protests. *Business Insider*. https://www.businessinsider.com/scientists-risk-arrest-in-global-climate-protests-2022-4?international=true&r=US&IR=T

Metsäranta, V. (2021). Eco-anxiety and its link to the everyday life choices of young Finns in 2020. *JYX Digital Repository*. https://jyx.jyu.fi/handle/123456789/76581?locale-attribute=en

Morrow, S. (2014). *Typhoen francisco scholarship repository*. Master's theses, p. 89. https://repository.usfca.edu/thes/89

Pereira, M., et al. (2015). *The relationship between connectedness to nature, environmental values, and pro-environmental behaviours*. Warwick Institute for Advanced Teaching and Learning (IATL). https://warwick.ac.uk/fac/cross_fac/iatl/reinvention/archive/volume8issue2/pereira

Philippine Commission on Women. (2020). *Environment sector*. GOVPH. https://pcw.gov.ph/environment/

Pihkala, P. (2018). Eco-anxiety, tragedy, and hope: Psychological and spiritual dimensions of climate change. *Wiley Online Library*. https://doi.org/10.1111/zygo.12407

Pihkala, P. (2020a). Anxiety and the ecological crisis: An analysis of eco-anxiety and climate anxiety. MDPI https://doi.org/10.3390/su12197836

Pihkala, P. (2020b). Eco-anxiety and environmental education. *Sustainability, 12*(23), 10149. https://doi.org/10.3390/su122310149

Reyes, M. E. S., et al. (2021). An investigation into the relationship between climate change anxiety and mental health among Gen Z Filipinos. *Current Psychology.* https://doi.org/10.1007/s12144-021-02099-3

Roberts, W., & Lauchlan, E. (2020). A world of worry: Exploring consumer eco-anxiety and environmental behaviours. *Shift Sustainability.* https://shift-sustainability.co.uk/wp-content/uploads/2020/10/Shift-Sustainability-World-of-Worry-consumer-environmental-climate-anxiety-October2020.pdf

Royal College of Psychiatrists. (2020). The climate crisis is taking a toll on the mental health of children and young people. *RC Psych.* https://www.rcpsych.ac.uk/news-and-features/latest-news/detail/2020/11/20/the-climate-crisis-is-taking-a-toll-on-the-mental-health-of-children-and-young-people?searchTerms=child%20psychiatrists%20survey

Searles, H. (1972). Unconscious processes in relation to the environmental crisis. *Psychoanalytic Review, 59*, 361.

Sulistyawati, S., et al. (2017). Assessment of knowledge regarding climate change and health among adolescents in Yogyakarta, Indonesia. *Hindawi Journal of Environmental and Public Health.* https://doi.org/10.1155/2018/9716831

UN Women. (2022). *Explainer: How gender inequality and climate change are interconnected.* UN Women. https://www.unwomen.org/en/news-stories/explainer/2022/02/explainer-how-gender-inequality-and-climate-change-are-interconnected

UNESCO. (2022). *Climate change education.* UNESCO. https://www.unesco.org/en/education/sustainable-development/climate-change

Whitcomb, I. G. (2021). Therapists are reckoning with eco-anxiety. *Scientific American.* https://www.scientificamerican.com/article/therapists-are-reckoning-with-eco

Whiting, K. (2021). Climate crisis: Eco-anxiety is growing in young people. *World Economic Forum.* https://www.weforum.org/agenda/2021/10/climate-crisis-eco-anxiety

World Health Organization. (2014). https://www.who.int/news/item/15-05-2014-world-health-statistics-2014

World Health Organization. (2021). Climate change and health. *WHO Health Topics.* https://www.who.int/news-room/fact-sheets/detail/climate-change-and-health

# Mental Health and Field Education Praxis During the COVID-19 Pandemic

**Meghan Boston-McKraken, Dionisio Nyaga, Rose Ann Torres, and Yashoda Fernando**

## Introduction

The COVID-19 pandemic had a profound effect on social work field education, presenting unique challenges to students, social work supervising field practicums supervisors, as well as field education coordinators and field stakeholders (Negi & E P, 2022). Available literature on social work field practicum (Fortune & Abramson, 1993; Petra et al., 2020; Panos et al., 2002) indicates that there is a gap on the topic of mental health among students, supervisors, and other stakeholders. In this regard, we attempt to bring forward the various unique mental health challenges and opportunities faced by these groups while undertaking field education/practicum. While there are various challenges that this demographic group faced, this paper seeks to pay attention to the question of mental health and the ways in which they negotiated themselves in the midst of the pandemic. This article explores the various challenges and opportunities that impact on mental health and well-being, creative solutions, and lessons learned during this unprecedented time.

M. Boston-McKraken · D. Nyaga (✉) · R. A. Torres · Y. Fernando
School of Social Work, Algoma University, Sault ste Marie, ON, Canada
e-mail: meghan.boston-mccracken@algomau.ca

© The Author(s), under exclusive license to Springer Nature Switzerland AG 2024    45
D. Nyaga, R. A. Torres (eds.), *Reimagining Mental Health and Addiction Under the Covid-19 Pandemic,* Volume 1, Advances in Mental Health and Addiction,
https://doi.org/10.1007/978-3-031-58367-4_5

## Literature Review

### *Challenges Prior to the COVID-19 Pandemic*

Field education programs are closely connected with health, community, and social services, where most field practicum opportunities are offered. Mental health as a social issue is pertinent in social work care, and yet those who provide care face it in disproportionate ways. In the context of neoliberal austerity measures (Baines, 2017), community agencies and organizations that supervise students are under increasing demands to provide social services with limited resources, making supervising practicum students increasingly unfeasible (Preston et al., 2014; Wiebe, 2010). Neoliberalism as a market rationality has affected social services in a myriad of ways among them being precarious jobs, cuts in social services, decreased worker morale, decreased number of social service workers, lack of unionization, worker fatigue, decreased advocacy, and many other challenges (Baines et al., 2022). This has had immense mental health challenges to care providers who must find ways to survive while simultaneously trying to supervise placement students. This has a fundamental effect on availability of placement spaces and overall placement students' field experience.

Field education in Canada has been in crisis for several years (Ayala et al., 2018), due to a number of factors such as increased student enrollments in Canada compared to available placement spaces (Regehr, 2013). Moreover, the increased focus on experiential learning and co-op in college and university settings has resulted in many education programs approaching the same organizations for limited field practicum opportunities (Ayala et al., 2018). This competition for practicum spaces by education programs brought about by neoliberalism was compounded by COVID-19 as many students tried to negotiate practicum spaces virtually while also dealing with their mental health.

The pandemic provided insights and challenges into the field education system. During the pandemic, social workers, students, and organizations in the field education system had to adapt quickly to new ways of working, particularly with the adoption of virtual technologies. Canadian universities and field offices rapidly shifted to virtual platforms during COVID-19, which impacted all aspects of social work programs, including field education (Canadian Association for Social Work Education [CASWE], 2020). COVID-19 amplified the already prevailing challenges in field education and introduced unique difficulties for students, staff, and organizations. Social workers had to rapidly adapt to new ways of working, such as using virtual technologies, resulting in a wide range of experiences. For example, Ashcroft et al. (2021) surveyed social workers who were members of a provincial social work association in Ontario, Canada. They found the transition to virtual care both challenging and beneficial.

This adaptation brought about a range of experiences, with both challenges and benefits, which remains connected to neoliberal economic agenda. Social workers faced heightened stressors, such as increased workloads, concerns for personal health and safety, and the complexities of managing personal well-being. Placement students experienced emotional tolls as they juggled remote or hybrid field practicums along with other responsibilities. The pandemic also revealed social disparities, with mothers disproportionately shouldering the burden of parenting and work, reporting higher levels of psychological distress. These experiences were compounded by factors such as race, gender, sexual orientation, disability, and citizenship among other social markers. There was a calculated erasure of emotions into care provision, and instead care was fundamentally rationalized, which made placement students face unequal burnouts as they try to negotiate themselves in care provision. Field coordinators and field teams faced the challenge of navigating COVID-19 protocols and supporting students in this new context while still trying to balance their personal protection from the pandemic.

In one of the studies done during the pandemic, participants reported fatigue related to the shift to virtual care, feelings of isolation, profound stress, a lack of work-life balance, and burnout (Ashcroft et al., 2021).

Many stressors emerged such as increased workload, adapting in-person services, concerns for personal health and safety, personal caregiving responsibilities, dealing with clients with increasing complexities, and managing personal well-being. Some social workers even experienced job losses or redeployment to new settings. These challenges faced by employees had immense effects on placement students in terms of their mental health and overall experiences in placement spots. Students experienced an emotional toll as they adapted to online learning and the demands to complete program requirements (Christensen et al., 2023). For example, many students were obligated to switch to remote or hybrid situations for their field practicums. Students who were single parents were disproportionately affected, as some had to balance caring for children attending school from home, sick family members, employment, coursework, and field practicum demands (Christensen et al., 2023). Other students who did their field practicums in essential services continued to go in-person but faced the additional stresses related to COVID-19 protocols and fears of exposing their families or communities to the virus. Field education coordinators and teams often faced the challenge of finding out COVID-19 protocols, communicating with community organizations, and relaying this information to students, which amplified the existing challenges and demands (Ossais et al., 2021).

The struggle of parenting and work disproportionately affected mothering students, who carried a unique heavier load in providing childcare during the COVID-19 crisis even while still working, reporting higher levels of psychological distress (Zamarro & Prados, 2021). The struggles become more complicated when the mothering students are racialized and Indigenous because they have to deal with the interlocking systems of oppression and marginalization. For example, an Asian student mother has to deal with anti-Asian sexism and racism, and a Black mother has to deal with anti-Black sexism and racism. These forms of oppression have contributed a great deal in performing their role as a mother and as a student.

## Theoretical Framework

Care as a human service has over time been violent and meant to mark some bodies as providers and saviors while others as receivers of arms. Those who receive are marked as subhuman while those who provide as saviors of the deplorables. This philosophical orientation continues to define the how of social work care provision where service users are marked as broken objects that need to be repaired to enter the human community. Such forms of repairs mark the receivers as wrong and immoral awaiting correction from their wrongdoing. This becomes even more compounded when care is provided virtually. The distance between the care provider and the receiver helps mark care provision as a rational process devoid of any emotions. Social distance provides a space for violence against those who receive service (this includes social work placement students) and perpetrated by those who provide care services.

Virtualization of care also meant students would not have an in-person practicum experience which translated to limited human connection. We would argue that such forms of virtualized care provided spaces of violence between student placement and agency and care receiver. This is not a new phenomenon only that COVID-19 compounded it in unique ways. Social work as a care profession has employed ethical standards to design ways in which to provide care in ways that are human, confidential, and ethical. While that is the case, such care provided in public spaces has been violent and meant to surveille social service users (Moffatt, 1999).

## Analysis

### *Opportunities in the Midst of Crisis*

Amid the COVID-19 pandemic, there were innovations in working together, exemplified by regular meetings of the *Alliance of Ontario Social Work Field Education Directors (AOSWFED)* and *the CASWE Field Education Committee.* These meetings provided the opportunity for information-sharing and support to respond to students and the new context of field education during the COVID-19 pandemic. Strategies and tactics to support students meet their placement plan such as flexibility, the reduction in field practicum hours permitted by the CASWE, and support for the remote completion of field practicum hours (e.g., Christensen et al., 2023) helped and provided opportunities for imagining placement and social work differently.

## Lessons Learned and Shaping the Future

Despite the challenges, the pandemic fostered innovations and collaboration within field education teams and the field education community. Regular meetings of organizations such as the Alliance of Ontario Social Work Field Education Directors (AOSWFED) and the CASWE Field Education Committee provided crucial support and information-sharing opportunities. Strategies to support students, such as flexibility in field hours and remote practicum options, aimed to enhance accessibility and meet the unique needs of students during these challenging times.

There is ongoing engagement around reduced field practicum hours and ensuring that the time students have is used for meaningful learning (Ossais et al., 2021). The flexibility and support for remote and hybrid field practicums increased accessibility for some students.

## Conclusion

The COVID-19 pandemic had a significant mental health impact on social work field education in Canada. Even before the pandemic, the field education system faced various challenges brought about by neoliberal agenda. Among those challenges were mental health issues that were faced by social work practitioners. This was compounded by COVID-19 wherein various stakeholders in the care profession had to find alternative ways to negotiate the challenges. The lessons learned during the pandemic offer insights and opportunities to reimagine the field education system to make it more resilient, responsive to future challenges, accessible, and inclusive. Collaboration, flexibility, and continued dialogue among stakeholders will be key in shaping the future of social work field education. By learning from the pandemic and building on the innovations, the field can strive to create a more inclusive and impactful learning environment for future social workers, better equipping them to address the evolving needs of communities and individuals for a more equitable and just society.

## References

Ashcroft, R., Sur, D., Greenblatt, A., & Donahue, P. (2021). The impact of the COVID-19 pandemic on social workers at the frontline: A survey of Canadian social workers. *British Journal of Social Work*, bcab158. https://doi.org/10.1093/bjsw/bcab158

Ayala, J., Drolet, J., Fulton, A., Hewson, J., Letkemann, L., Baynton, M., Elliot, G., Judge-Stasiak, A., Blaug, C., Tetreault, A. G., & Schweizer, E. (2018). Field education in crisis: Experiences of field education coordinators in Canada. *Social Work Education, 37*(3), 281–293. https://doi.org/10.1080/02615479.2017.1397109

Baines, D. (Ed.). (2017). Doing anti-oppressive practice: social justice social work (3rd edition.). Fernwood Publishing.

Baines, D., Clark, N., & Bennett, B. (2022). *Doing anti-oppressive social work: rethinking theory and practice* (D. Baines, N. Clark, & B. Bennett, Eds.; 4th ed.). Fernwood Publishing.

Canadian Association of Social Work Education. (2020, March 18). *COVID-19 communication: Field education placements*. CASWE-ACFTS. https://caswe-acfts.ca/covid-19-communication-field-education-placements/

Christensen, M., Gamble, J., & Morrow, D. F. (2023). Preliminary findings on long-term impacts of the COVID-19 pandemic on social work students. *Journal of Teaching in Social Work, 43*(2), 175–192. https://doi.org/10.1080/08841233.2023.2176016

Fortune, A. E., & Abramson, J. S. (1993). Predictors of satisfaction with field practicum among social work students. *The Clinical Supervisor, 11*(1), 95–110. https://doi.org/10.1300/J001v11n01_07.    https://www.proquest.com/docview/2583946092/abstract/5680359157EC45D0PQ/1

Moffatt, K. (1999). Surveillance and government of the the welfare recipient. In A. Chambon, A. Irving, & L. Epstein (Eds.), *Reading Foucault for social work* (pp. 219–242). New York, NY: Columbia University Press.

Negi, D. P., & E P, A. A. (2022). "Neither it had social work components nor experiential": Students' perspectives of online fieldwork practice during COVID-19 in India. *Asian Social Work and Policy Review, 16*(3), 237–245. https://doi.org/10.1111/aswp.12262

Ossais, J., Drolet, J., Alemi, M. I., Collins, T., Au, C., Bogo, M., Charles, G., Franco, M., Henton, J., Huang, L. X., Kaushik, V., McConnell, S., Nicholas, D., Shenton, H., Sussman, T., Walsh, C., & Wickman, J. (2021). Canadian social work field education during a global pandemic: A comparison of student and field instructor perspectives. *Journal of Comparative Social Work, 16*(2), Article 2. https://doi.org/10.31265/jcsw.v16i2.406

Panos, P. T., Panos, A., Cox, S. E., Roby, J. L., & Matheson, K. W. (2002). Ethical issues concerning the use of videoconferencing to supervise international social work field practicum students. *Journal of Social Work Education, 38*(3), 421–437. https://doi.org/10.1080/10437797.2002.10779108

Petra, M. M., Tripepi, S., & Guardiola, L. (2020). How many hours is enough? The effects of changes in field practicum hours on student preparedness for social work. *Field Educator, 10*(1), 1–21, see https://fieldeducator.simmons.edu/wp-content/uploads/2020/05/20-235-1.pdf

Preston, S., George, P., & Silver, S. (2014). Field education in social work: The need for reimagining. *Critical Social Work, 15*(1). Retrieved from http://www1.uwindsor.ca/criticalsocialwork/

Regehr, C. (2013). Trends in higher education in Canada and implications for social work education. *Social Work Education: The International Journal, 32*(6), 700–714. https://doi.org/10.1080/02615479.2013.785798

Wiebe, M. (2010). Pushing the boundaries of the social work practicum: Rethinking sites and supervision toward radical practice. *Journal of Progressive Human Services, 21*(1), 66–82. https://doi.org/10.1080/10428231003782517

Zamarro, G., & Prados, M. J. (2021). Gender differences in couples' division of childcare, work and mental health during COVID-19. *Review of Economics of the Household, 19*(1), 11–40. https://doi.org/10.1007/s11150-020-09534-7

# Supporting Ontario's Consumer/Survivor Initiatives and Their Importance to the Ontario Community Mental Health and Addictions System During the COVID-19 Pandemic

**Tanya Shute and Allyson Theodorou**

In the early 1990s, the Ontario government established a different kind of mental health organization called Consumer/Survivor Initiatives (CSIs), a kind of consumer/survivor-run organization mandated to be governed independently by people who identified as consumers/survivors of the mental health system. Operating on the principles of self-help and mutual aid, CSIs function as low-barrier and quick-access alternatives to the mainstream mental health system. From the outset, approximately 40 CSIs were funded by the Ontario Ministry of Health and Long-Term Care (OMHLTC). Owing to a variety of factors, currently only seven or eight CSIs retain their independence, with the rest either closing their doors or amalgamated into flow-through arrangements with mainstream, non-consumer/survivor-led mental health organizations. The term consumer/survivor organizations (CSOs) will be used herein as a broad term to describe any consumer/survivor-led or governed organization (independent or otherwise). The following paper reports on some of the findings from a small-scale, qualitative inquiry into the data collection practices of CSOs in Ontario. Data collection in any social service organization is vital in order to be able to demonstrate to funders and the community that programs are effective and valuable to maintain sustainable funding. This is also true for CSOs, who are less well-known than other types of community mental health organizations and face greater challenges in terms of funding sustainability. This study into data collection practices in CSOs was undertaken to better understand the current data collection practices, which tend to be minimal in these organizations owing to their small infrastructure and budgets. This approach to data collection, although

T. Shute (✉)
School of Social Work, Laurentian University, Sudbury, ON, Canada
e-mail: tg_shute@laurentian.ca

A. Theodorou
PeerWorks, Toronto, ON, Canada

© The Author(s), under exclusive license to Springer Nature Switzerland AG 2024     51
D. Nyaga, R. A. Torres (eds.), *Reimagining Mental Health and Addiction Under the Covid-19 Pandemic,* Volume 1, Advances in Mental Health and Addiction,
https://doi.org/10.1007/978-3-031-58367-4_6

necessary, poses challenges for establishing empirically their effectiveness in the community mental health system. Because the inquiry was conducted during the early months of the pandemic, its challenges for these organizations became part of our conversations. As such, this chapter reports on some of the findings of this project as well as describes briefly CSOs' unique approach to the pandemic in these low-barrier/quick access peer support organizations in order to bring greater awareness about these unique organizations and the factors that contribute to a minimal approach to data collection practices.

## Brief Literature Review

Mutual aid and peer support have been the cornerstone of the consumer/survivor movement in Canada since widespread deinstitutionalization in the 1970s and 1980s. Developed out of necessity as an alternative to inadequate services in community, the success of peer-led mutual aid eventually led to the development of CSOs in Ontario (Trainor & Reville, 2014; Trainor et al., 1997). Diverse in character, CSOs come in the form of drop-in centers or social programming spaces and offer a variety of peer-based programming and support as well as access to survival needs. In 2004, legislation was changed to allow for non-consumer/survivor governance over these organizations and, as a result, only a handful retain their independence (Trainor & Reville, 2014).

Owing perhaps to a lack of awareness of these organizations in the broader academic community, research into the effectiveness of CSOs primarily reflects the 1990s/2000s when they were first developed and shows significant effectiveness as alternatives to hospital and crisis services in reduction of use and significant improvements in quality of life for participants (Canadian Mental Health Association, et al., 2005). A systematic review of consumer-led services found that users reported greater personal life satisfaction and fewer hospitalizations (Simpson & O'House, 2002). Doughty and Tse's (2011) integrative review also confirmed reductions in hospitalizations for CSO users. Nelson et al. (2007), in an Ontario-based study, found that after participating in a CSO for 18 months, CSO users had significantly greater reductions in hospitalizations, reductions in symptoms, improvements in social support, and quality of life compared to the control group. An early study done in Ontario's CSOs established that prior to joining a CSO, study participants had a mean number of 48.36 in-patient hospital days, and a mean number of 3.54 contacts with crisis services, which dropped to 4.29 inpatient use days and their crisis services use, dropped to a mean of 0.81 after participating in a CSO (Trainor et al., 1997). In an Ontario study, Forchuk et al. (2005) determined that peer mentorship from a CSO related to an earlier discharge from hospital of 116 days, translating into a $12 million savings to the healthcare system as a result of shorter hospital stays. Although shorter stays in not perhaps in the best interest of users, cost-effectiveness of interventions is a strong rationale for funding support. At 3-year follow-up, active participants had higher community integration and quality of life and scored lower on mental health symptom distress (Nelson et al., 2007). CSOs have been found to also decrease stigma of service use, and ensure consumer/survivor participation on a systems level (Janzen et al., 2006). Unfortunately, to the best of our knowledge, there has been no further experimental research published about the effectiveness of Ontario CSOs since the early 1990s and late 2000s.

Despite this promising effectiveness, CSOs receive inadequate and disproportionate funding compared to other mainstream community and hospital programs, putting significant pressure on effectiveness and sustainability (Doughty & Tse, 2011; O'Hagan et al., 2009; Tannenbaum, 2011). Combined with a lack of current evidence that can re-establish their approach and services as promising, this problem was the basis of the current study.

## Methodology

The current study was guided by the question: What are the current data collection practices undertaken in Ontario CSOs? Purposive convenience sampling was employed, with leaders contacted from a list of PeerWorks member organizations. From the list of potential leaders who expressed their willingness to participate, participants were selected based on the represented various organization forms CSOs currently take in Ontario: five were CSIs (independent CSOs), four were in flow-through/amalgamated arrangements with non-CSOs, and two were alternative businesses. The minimal inclusion criteria were that the leaders were in a management or executive position and could speak to the data collection approaches and procedures for their organizations. This SSHRC-funded project employed a qualitative approach, collecting data through semi-structured conversational interviews with 11 CSO leaders across Ontario, remotely conducted during the first year of the pandemic.

Qualitative data was transcribed using NVivo software and thematically analyzed by the principal investigator. Early findings were reviewed with many CSO leaders at the annual general meeting of PeerWorks member organizations in 2021.

## Findings and Discussion

What became clear was that data collection in many CSOs is based on the minimum character of data required by funders for accountability purposes, usually in the form of numbers of individuals served or attending a program and frequency of use counts. This is contextualized by the following contributing factors: (1) these organizations are under-resourced, (2) their ethic of peer support prioritizes all staff and assets toward service delivery, and (3) the pandemic presented new challenges for service delivery, and user/frequency counts are the simplest form of reporting accountability they can manage in this context. For the sake of brevity, one to two quotes will be used to demonstrate the spirit of these findings. More fulsome reporting on the findings is forthcoming.

CSOs are some of the most under-resourced of all community mental health organizations in Ontario and are unable to commit resources to data collection and evaluation:

> The amount of administration required, the technology required, the expertise… we would need to get extra funding…it would change us.. It gets so farther and farther away from people, and their connections with people. (CSI leader #1)

Being led and staffed by people with lived experience of mental health distress, the mental health system, problematic substance abuse, and homelessness, people work in these settings out of an orientation toward mutual aid. Administrative duties pull the few workers these organizations have away from their peers, and there are no administrative staff to fill in these duties. The result is, people are prioritized, not administrative tasks. With so little funding, all workers are direct service workers:

> We have two managers and 60-70 employees. The cost of that sparse budget is poverty wages for our staff We have a lot of good intentions [to collect better data], we have a hard time fulfilling them, because we're really spread – too little butter over too much bread… that scraping? That's us. (CSO leader #2)

When resources are tight, these organizations prioritize people over functions such as more robust service data collection beyond the minimum required for funding accountability:

> When people come in for peer support, they don't expect to sit down and have that peer do an intake or a whole bunch of forms. That's not what a peer relationship is. (CSO leader #4)

> …part of the work that we do is about not asking our users these kinds of questions [suicide risk] but we have to have this kind of data to support the value of our programs. You have to collect enough data to keep funders off your back, but not enough to scare away clients or lose sight of our approach in CSIs. It's a dance. (CSI leader #1)

Prioritizing people served over administrative needs only heightened during the pandemic. CSO leaders noted that they have the same administrative and reporting requirements as other larger, more resourced community mental health organizations, and to fulfill those obligations requires administrative infrastructure such as back-office supports. All leaders talked about needing to do more or better data collection, but that when the pandemic occurred, any and all resources and energy had to be redirected to the increased service need. Most community mental health organizations in Ontario received additional funds to resource the pandemic transition, but CSOs were not provided any additional funding, putting incredible pressure on already stretched budgets. CSO leaders said they just did the minimum data collection and could not implement any administrative changes/improvements during the past few years:

> There is a lot of pressure to do things like intakes or needs assessments, but we just don't have the infrastructure or the money to get the infrastructure…We didn't get any extra money to deal with the changes the pandemic brought, so there is even less money now than before to commit to anything but service priorities. (CSO leader #7)

## Responding to Pandemic Lockdown

To demonstrate the prioritizing of people over organizations in CSOs, confirmed by these interviews with CSO leaders during the early months of pandemic lockdown and by polling CSO workers and leaders at their provincial annual conference, no CSO in Ontario suspended services even temporarily in the early days of the lockdown. In the spirit of peer support and mutual aid, staff and volunteers went "old school," for example, setting up phone support trees or bus carpools organized to visit people outside residences. Because many of these organizations already offered some form of telephone support, some offered it 24 h a day. Care packages were prepared for "drop-by" instead of drop-in visitors who rely on these organizations for survival supplies. As low-barrier, quick-access organizations with no intakes or wait lists, new users were supported in some way the very same day they reached out. These kinds of mutual aid are most easily captured using the user/frequency counts approach employed by CSOs but cannot capture the full story of the effect on users.

This minimalist approach to service data collection is both necessary and functional in terms of serving the unique nonclinical nature of CSO work. Given the growing acuity of need in the mental health sector, exacerbated by the unforeseen chaos caused by the COVID-19 pandemic, these peer support/mutual aid organizations cannot abandon their peers out of lack of resources, divert funds away from their service needs, or prioritize data and research concerns under such conditions.

## Conclusion and Implications for Social Work Practice

The study findings reveal CSOs in Ontario face unique challenges and limitations to their ability to collect the data to establish their current evidence base for their approach. Participants all revealed being hired for lived expertise (and not for administrative or executive experience or education) which means that people who work in CSOs embody the spirit peer support and mutual aid and administrative tasks must not overshadow their unique approach. Also, as under-resourced organizations compared to their non-CSO community mental health counterparts, they do not have back-office departments or administrative employees, with all staff providing front-line supports, including executive directors. CSO leaders were aware that their current approach to data collection was limited and that there was pressure to be able to provide more robust data to demonstrate their value in Ontario's mental health system.

CSOs require infrastructure and resources to better capture service-use data that aligns with their unique approach and needs to remain low-barrier/quick access. Most existing systems are large and expensive, require a lot of training, and are clinically focused, so hardly practical for CSOs. Without an infusion of resources forthcoming, the sector needs help to develop tailored data collection approaches and tools. Social workers can help by raising awareness about CSOs in their communities and developing collaborative participatory program evaluation projects—but without expecting CSOs to provide resources at all. As the academic research about CSIs has fallen off since their inception (1990s to mid-2000s), social work researchers are positioned well to work in collaborative, participatory action, "nothing about us, without us" ways that are the heart of the CSO sector and can support CSOs to tell their current story, strengthening their uncertain future in the community mental health and addictions system in Ontario.

# References

Canadian Mental Health Association, Centre for Addiction and Mental Health, Ontario Federation of Community Mental Health and Addictions Programs, and Ontario Peer Development Initiatives. (2005). *Consumer survivor initiatives: Impacts, outcomes and effectiveness.* Retrieved from: https://ontario.cmha.ca/wp-content/uploads/2005/03/cmha_ontario_consumer_survivor_initiatives_2005.pdf

Doughty, C., & Tse, S. (2011). Can consumer-led mental health services be equally effective? An integrative review of CLMH services in high-income countries. *Community Mental Health Journal, 47,* 252–266. https://doi.org/10.1007/s10597-010-9321-5

Forchuk, C., Martin, M. L., Chan, Y. L., & Jensen, E. (2005). Therapeutic relationships: From psychiatric hospital to community. *Journal of Psychiatric Mental Health Nursing, 12*(5), 556–564.

Janzen, R., Nelson, G., Trainor, J., & Ochocka, J. (2006). A longitudinal study of mental health consumer/survivor initiatives: Part 4 benefits beyond the self? A quantitative and qualitative study of system-level activities and impacts. *Journal of Community Psychology, 34*(3), 285–303. https://doi.org/10.1002/jcop.20100

Nelson, G., Ochocka, J., Janzen, R., Trainor, J., Goering, P., & Lamotey, J. (2007). A longitudinal study of mental health consumer/survivor initiatives: Part V outcomes at a 3-year follow-up. *Journal of Community Psychology, 35*(5). https://doi.org/10.1002/jcop.20171

O'Hagan, M., McKee, H., & Priest, R. (2009, June). Consumer/survivor initiatives in Ontario: Building for an equitable future. Ontario Federation of Community Mental Health and Addictions Programs. Retrieved from: http://www.maryohagan.com/resources/Peer%20Services%20in%20Ontario.pdf

Simpson, E. L., & O'House, A. (2002). Involving users in the delivery and evaluation of mental health services: Systematic review. *BMJ, 325.* Retrieved from: https://www.bmj.com/content/bmj/325/7375/1265.full.pdf

Tannenbaum, S. J. (2011). Characteristics associated with organizational independence in consumer-operated service organizations. *Psychiatric Rehabilitation Journal, 34*(3), 248–251.

Trainor, J., & Reville, D. (2014). Beginning to take control: Ontario's consumer/survivor development initiative. In G. Nelson, B. Kloos, & J. Ornelas (Eds.), *Community psychology and community mental health: Towards transformative change* (pp. 309–326). Oxford Academic. Retrieved from: https://doi.org/10.1093/acprof:oso/9780199362424.003.0015

Trainor, J., Shepherd, M., Boydell, K. M., Leff, A., & Crawford, E. (1997). Beyond the service paradigm: The impact and implications of consumer/survivor initiatives. *Psychiatric Rehabilitation Journal, 21,* 132–140.

# Setting Them Up for Success: The School System and Children's Mental Health

Sidney T. Wilson

## Setting Them Up for Success: The School System and Children MH

Mental health—although not a new concept—is the topic of many conversations currently. There is a mental health crisis within our society. If we want to see a bright future, it is important that we work toward prevention and intervention at a young age. There is a common idea that children are resilient. When they break bones, it's easier for the bones to heal than those of an adult. Society puts this idea onto their mental health as well. When a child faces hardship, we admire their resilience. The fact is children should not have to be resilient. This is especially true when it comes to school. School is meant to be a safe space—a place where children learn, play, and spend most of their childhood which should be somewhere that fosters setting kids up for success. It seems these days that schools are setting them up for failure instead. Whether it is the effects of the pandemic, the expectations, the physical classroom, or the curriculum, something is working against the children.

For this paper, I have read a variety of articles that look into different areas of schools/school culture and the education system.

S. T. Wilson (✉)
School of Social Work, Algoma University, Sault ste Marie, ON, Canada
e-mail: swilson@algomau.ca

© The Author(s), under exclusive license to Springer Nature Switzerland AG 2024
D. Nyaga, R. A. Torres (eds.), *Reimagining Mental Health and Addiction Under the Covid-19 Pandemic,* Volume 1, Advances in Mental Health and Addiction,
https://doi.org/10.1007/978-3-031-58367-4_7

## Children's Mental Health

It is vital that we prioritize children's mental health. While their brains are still developing, children's emotional well-being can severely impact their future. According to the Mental Health Commission of Canada, roughly 1.2 million children within Canada are living with a mental illness (2021). That number does not include those children who are facing mental health challenges that are not considered to be a diagnosable mental illness. These challenges can be influenced by a variety of factors. Some of those factors are poverty, academics, food insecurity, family dynamics, and peer relationships. Within the last decade, there has been a concerning rise in emergency department (ED) visits from children and youth regarding their mental health (Chiu et al., 2020). In an article written by Chiu et al., data is reviewed from the Ontario Mental Health Reporting System (OMHRS) in order to gain a better understanding of the rise in ED visits (2020). The authors also delve into the possible influencing factors that contribute to the rise in mental health-related visits.

The study of the OMHRS found that there has been a significant increase in mental health-related visits to the ED among children aged 5–24 years old, with the authors noting the sharpest rise among girls aged 10–17 (Chiu et al., 2020). A limitation of this study is the concept of gender—as the article used information collected from valid health cards, they were limited to female and male as gender options (Chiu et al., 2020). Therefore, there is a lack of information surrounding transgendered, two-spirited, and other gender identities. One area in which this article did look deeper into was the concept of rural versus urban. In rural communities, the number of mental health-related ED visits were higher (Chiu et al., 2020). Within smaller/rural communities, there are often less resources available, especially quick response and non-referral resources (Chiu et al., 2020). Further into this paper, I will discuss the importance of mental health resources being available within the school system in order to fill this gap.

## Curriculum/Standardized Testing

Within Ontario, in order to evaluate the effectiveness of education, the Educational Quality and Accountability Office (EQAO) was created (Jang & Sinclair, 2018). To assess Ontario's curriculum and education delivery, standardized testing is implemented during "grades 3, 6, 9, and 10" (Jang & Sinclair, 2018, p. 2). These tests were developed in hopes of determining if the education system was implemented with equality and equity (Jang & Sinclair, 2018). Society called for a way to maintain that every child was getting a "basic education" (Jang & Sinclair, 2018, p. 5). However, there are some flaws within the system. In Ontario, the test given in grade 10 is a determining factor for graduation. If a student fails this exam, they must either retake the test or enroll in a yearlong literacy/language class (Jang & Sinclair,

2018). Knowing that this test impacts your ability to graduate can cause unnecessary stress to what are already stressful times (adolescence). This is extremely important to consider when looking at children from lower socioeconomic backgrounds, racialized groups, or children who are facing ongoing multiple stressors. A study done in 2018 looked at cortisol levels in students on an average school week versus exam week (National Bureau of Economic Research, Inc., 2018). It showed that on average, cortisol levels were higher than normal during exam week. This may be a positive thing; however, cortisol provides a boost of energy and motivation to act accordingly when faced with a challenge (National Bureau of Economic Research, Inc., 2018). However, the response to the heightened level of cortisol differed based on those impacted by poverty (housing insecurity, food insecurity, etc.), racialized oppression, and trauma/mental health challenges (abuse, major illness, ADHD, anxiety, etc.). When children are continuously facing these challenges, their reactions to higher levels of cortisol may result in a state of hyperarousal (difficulty concentrating and self-regulating, etc.). This can negatively impact the outcomes of their tests. Although many of these tests are not used to determine grades, the pressure to achieve higher success can be detrimental to one's self-esteem, which is something that I have seen firsthand while working as a CYW and EA.

When it comes to the curriculum, the impacts of colonialism are still prevalent, and these can have a negative impact on Indigenous children attending public school (Miles, 2021). Within Canada it is mandatory for students to complete Social Studies/History to graduate. The students learn what is deemed the history of Canada. However, the history of Canada and Indigenous peoples is lacking in detail. At this point, it is important to address the horrifying truth behind how the settlers of Canada treated Indigenous peoples, specifically the children. For over 100 years, children were removed from their homes and sent to live in residential schools. These schools were operated by Catholic or Christian churches. The parents were forced to sign over their custodial rights to the church or face terrible consequences (Starblanket et al., 2020). Within these so-called schools, children were beaten, raped, neglected, and forced to abandon their culture and identities (Starblanket et al., 2020). This has led to intergenerational trauma that is still seen today. Yet, our Social Studies/History textbooks barely touch on this subject. In 2015, the Truth and Reconciliation Commission of Canada (TRC) released a report that listed 94 calls to action, one of which is directed specifically toward the education system—the request for curriculums to address the truth behind Canada's history of residential schooling (Miles, 2021). It was made apparent just how little is taught about the residential schools when news of the unmarked graves being found on residential school property broke (Miles, 2021). Society was shocked to hear that children were treated with such callous disregard. Not acknowledging the truth about residential schools is a systemic way of telling an entire culture that they are not important. This historic denial also subconsciously teaches non-Indigenous children that Indigenous people and culture are not important. This keeps systemic and direct racism strong.

Another way in which racism within the curriculum may impact children's mental health is seen within the English courses. When we look at the literature that students are reading for class, we often see European/white authors. We see people like Shakespeare and Jane Austin; we rarely see Indigenous authors. The authors chosen are subject to change from teacher to teacher. There are some teachers who make a conscious choice to incorporate a diverse reading list; however, that is not the norm. This is also true for students within the LGBTQ2+ community. With little to no representation, it is easy for children and youth to feel isolated. This is something that author Shawna Carroll writes strongly about in her article written in 2018. Although her article focuses on a feminist perspective, she discusses how colonialism created and influenced the lack of diversity within the school curriculum (Carroll, 2018).

## COVID-19

Due to the spread of a virus known as COVID-19, many schools across Canada closed their doors for large chunks of time. Students and staff were forced to stay home and work within the virtual world. Approximately 5.7 million students within Canada were impacted by COVID-19's closing of the schools (Vaillancourt et al., 2021). In Ontario, during March 2020 desks had to be a certain amount of space apart from each other, and nothing physical was to be shared. Gone were the days of "sharing is caring." There was already anxiety in the air as students and staff feared getting sick. Things only got worse from there. Staff and students alike felt the weight of uncertainty as the pandemic spread and talks of lockdowns began. When the schools were told to close and switch to virtual classrooms, many issues became apparent (Vaillancourt et al., 2021).

One area in which children and youth were negatively impacted by COVID-19 was their mental health (Vaillancourt et al., 2021). For some students, school is the majority of their social interactions. It can be where they find their sense of belonging (friend groups, extracurricular school clubs, academics, etc.). The pandemic denied students the ability to have face to face, in-person interactions. This isolation had negative consequences (Vaillancourt et al., 2021). A study focusing on Ontario students (elementary and secondary) showed that during the school closures, many students reported higher rates of sadness, loneliness, and anxiety (both related and unrelated to the pandemic) (Vaillancourt et al., 2021).

Schools provide a variety of resources for students. As mentioned above, friends can play a large role in one's mental health, but there are also many adults within the school system who support the students as well. For some students, teachers, support staff, and administrators help to support children's mental health. These adults not only provide a safe person for children and youth to trust, but they also can be an advocate for these children. In some cases, home life is unsafe. Some children face violence/abuse within the home. School is typically where these events get reported (Vaillancourt et al., 2021). The closure of schools resulted in staff being unable to support these particular students, in some cases placing the children at risk due to spending more time at home—not to mention the added stress that COVID-19 put on families.

For students with learning disabilities, English as a second language, or those needing a bit more support, these closures not only impacted their education but also their self-esteem. During the pandemic, I worked at a mental health day treatment program (a program that mimicked school structure). When things switched to virtual learning/treatment, it was incredibly challenging for both students and staff. For myself, it was challenging to learn how to use technology while supporting my clients. For my clients (the students), not only did they have to learn how to do their work online, but they also had the added challenge of learning while struggling with their mental health and learning challenges. I saw how this played a role in harming their self-esteem. On top of the struggles with learning from home, many students (my clients included) struggled without the structure and support that the classroom provided them.

## School/Classroom Culture and the Physical Space

The physical environment can play a large role in one's mental health and ability to succeed. When we think about the classroom, we typically think about wooden desks and hard chairs in rows facing the black/whiteboard. This has been the case for many years. In the younger grades (k-8) fixed seating is common. Fixed seating is where the teacher decides the type of seat the student sits in and where they sit. There are pros and cons to fixed seating. Some of the positives are helping a student make positive choices, eliminating distractions, and reducing conflict. However, some of the negatives can be the furniture contributing to ableism, lack of autonomy, and lack of comfort (both physically and mentally). From personal experience, fixed seating can hinder one's ability to learn. As a plus-sized individual with a chronic pain disorder, sitting at a desk, in a hard, plastic chair was often the bane of my existence. I could not concentrate on what I was learning due to the discomfort I was experiencing. This was also an issue due to my sensory issues (due to being on the autism spectrum disorder). Later in this paper, I will discuss the benefits of flexible seating to address this concern.

More research needs to be done on the topic of the physical environment; however, I have witnessed a variety of situations in which changing the environment has benefited the student. This also crosses over into classroom culture. It is a common practice for schools and classrooms to follow the fixed seating culture. When I am working within schools, supporting students with a variety of needs, a common issue I witness is the idea that the student needs to sit at their desk and be quiet. This can be extremely challenging for some students. Students with attention deficit hyperactivity disorder (ADHD) may find sitting on stationary for prolonged periods of time to be challenging. Even students (especially the younger students) without ADHD may find sitting at a desk very challenging.

Another way in which classroom culture can negatively affect students' well-being is through staff and student relationships. While working within schools, I have seen a diverse group of teachers. I have had the pleasure of working with teachers who focus on a strength-based approach and are known for hyping up every student they teach. I unfortunately have also worked with teachers who are the opposite. Their negativity oozes out of them and impacts how they treat their students. In an article written by Andrew J. Hill and Daniel B. Jones, the concept of self-fulfilling prophecies created by teachers is discussed (2021). This paper focuses on how the negative interactions and expectations put on students by teachers can guide how successful the student is in the future. This can also impact their mental health and well-being. The article suggests that if a young student is faced with negative expectations and negative teacher-student relationships, they will live up to those expectations (Hill & Jones, 2021). Some students internalize the negativity, and it becomes their reality (Hill & Jones, 2021).

I personally experienced a negative student-teacher relationship when I was younger. When I was struggling with academics, I was met with jokes about my intelligence, annoyed body language, and hostility when I asked questions. Eventually, I withdrew from engaging with the teacher and the class. This resulted in me failing a class that was mandatory for me to pass. My experience was mild compared to some students. The article mentioned above spoke about the experience of black students and the different expectations put on them than their white classmates (Hill & Jones, 2021). Simply based on the color of their skin, the teachers in this particular study had lower academic expectations for them (Hill & Jones, 2021). When the person who is supposed to be helping you become the best possible does not think that you are capable of being the best, it is not hard to understand why this becomes a self-fulfilling prophecy.

## How Can We Change

It is evident that something is not working within our educational system. Schools are in a crisis and the needs of the generations coming up are not being met. So, the question is, how can we change the system to support these kids? This section of the paper will discuss some current changes that are being made such as flexible seating, teaching to the student versus the curriculum, and incorporating mental health services within the school system. Although these are changes that are being made, they are still not the norm. There needs to be more exploration into the changes we can make and how to make them.

## *Mental Health Services Within Schools*

An article written by Hoover and Bostic discusses the importance of having access to in school mental health services (2021). As I discussed earlier within this paper, children and youth are currently facing a mental health crisis. Finding and accessing mental health services within a community can be extremely challenging and over-whelming for families. This can be due to a variety of factors such as lack of resources, poverty, and even lack of knowledge (Hoover & Bostic, 2021). By incor-porating more mental health services within the school system, some of the barriers could be addressed.

Children and youth spend the majority of their time at school. Most schools have free transportation to and from school which eliminates the stress of finding trans-portation (Hoover & Bostic, 2021). Although accessing these services would involve the student's educational day being interrupted, the long-term effects of accessing mental health services would outweigh the negative. Some students are in such a crisis that their brains are in survival mode. Therefore, they likely are not actually learning as much as they could be.

Having the services within the school can also be more comfortable for the child (Hoover & Bostic, 2021). Talking about challenging subjects can be extremely chal-lenging. Add being in a new environment with a stranger, and it might be even more challenging. If these services were within the school, students may feel safer and more comfortable. It can also allow the service providers to be a familiar face within the school. Students may feel more comfortable meeting with the providers if they have seen them continuously within the school (Hoover & Bostic, 2021).

This would also allow for supporting staff (teachers, educational assistants, and administrators) to have an ongoing working relationship with the mental health ser-vice providers (Hoover & Bostic, 2021). In order to fully support these children, continuity of care is important. Having teachers and support staff in the same build-ing as the students' mental health service providers would allow for the team to meet and plan with ease (Hoover & Bostic, 2021). Brief check-ins and discussions can also be done as everyone is in the same building.

## *Teaching to the Child, Not the Curriculum*

When a child has autonomy within their education, they are more likely to engage with the course materials, a concept explored by Nancy Barile, a teacher in the USA (Chiles, 2019). When met with the challenge of a student who would not complete any homework, Barile asked what they could do to support them. The end result of that conversation led to Barile creating an English class that was inspired by AMC's "The Walking Dead" while still meeting the curriculum's guidelines—the results were outstanding (Chiles, 2019).

When the school looked at the productivity of the students attending Barile's class, the changes were clear. The level of engagement within class went up, and the quality of work submitted was increased (Chiles, 2019). The article written about this particular class also mentioned how the students who took this class were more likely to enroll in university-level senior English class than those who did not take the specialized class (Chiles, 2019).

So, what does this mean? Well, it means that students are more likely to positively engage with their education when they have autonomy around how they learn. When students are positively engaged with their education, their well-being reflects that.

## *The Physical Space and School Culture*

As I discussed above, the physical environment of a classroom can have an impact on how successful the students are. Some suggest that classrooms should explore the concept of flexible seating (Bluteau et al., 2022). Flexible seating involves a variety of options of where to sit and how to "be" within the classroom (Bluteau et al., 2022). Some ways to incorporate flexible seating into the classroom are through providing a variety of furniture, and Bluteau advocates the use of cushions, bouncy balls, couches, and mats as alternative seating arrangements (2022).

When a child is developing, autonomy is important for well-being. Allowing a child to pick where they sit and on what type of furniture (flexible seating) can allow the student to feel in charge of their own body and learning (Bluteau et al., 2022). Flexible seating can also help to learn and strengthen self-regulation, adaptability, and problem-solving skills. Self-regulation, adaptability, and problem-solving skills are all crucial for an individual's mental well-being. Classrooms that have flexible seating reported that the students were more engaged, calm, and positive when in the classroom (Bluteau et al., 2022).

By incorporating flexible seating, the classroom can also become more accessible. Had I, as a child, had different options of seating, I may have been able to focus more and engage in my education. For students who struggle to sit still, having seats that promote movement can help them stay engaged and focused versus getting frustrated trying to sit still. When the classroom is more accessible, more students feel welcome and comfortable in the environment. This helps to promote positive well-being.

When it comes to school culture, one of the most impactful ways in which we can change is through alternative learning. Not only does this address physical space, but it also addresses how we view learning and the curriculum. For example, there are a few different alternative learning options within Canada. One of these options is land-based learning (Samuel Centre for Social Connectedness, n.d.). Land-based learning can look different depending on the program. Within Canada, there are a few Indigenous focused land-based learning programs. Land-based learning uses Indigenous knowledge and ways of learning to teach both cultural traditional living and Western curriculum (Samuel Centre for Social Connectedness, n.d.). Learning from and interacting with the land has many benefits. Not only does it allow students to be physically moving and interacting, but it also promotes a healthy relationship with the environment, the community, and one's self (Samuel Centre for Social Connectedness, n.d.). Learning about Indigenous culture and traditions from elders allows for Indigenous children and youth to connect with their culture and identity which can positively impact one's mental health. The Western education model could benefit from incorporating some values and practices that land-based learning programs focus on.

## Conclusion

It is evident that children and youth within Canada are struggling as there is a rise in mental health concerns (Mental Health Commission of Canada, 2021). When discussing children and youth, it only makes sense to examine the impact that the school system has on their mental well-being. Children spend the majority of their time within school. Testing, the curriculum, COVID-19, school/classroom culture, and the physical environment affect children every day. It is time that something changed in order to support the next generations of leaders.

**Acknowledgements** I acknowledge my experiences as a neurodivergent individual, and my views on this subject are inspired by my own personal experiences. My work as a Child and Youth Worker and Educational Assistant also impacts how I view the education system. I acknowledge that I, as a settler on this land, have views that are influenced by colonialism. Being a white, educated, cis-female puts me in a position of privilege. It is important that I am aware of this while discussing oppression of any kind.

## References

Bluteau, J., Aubenas, S., & Dufour, F. (2022). Influence of flexible classroom seating on the well-being and mental health of upper elementary school students: A gender analysis. *Frontiers in Psychology, 13*, 2493.

Carroll, S. M. (2018). Uncovering white settler colonial discourse in curricula with anticolonial feminism. *Journal of Curriculum Theorizing, 33*(1), 22–39.

Chiles, N. (2019). Teaching to the student, not the test. *The Education Digest, 84*(8), 26–32.

Chiu, M., Gatov, E., Fung, K., Kurdyak, P., & Guttmann, A. (2020). Deconstructing the rise in mental health-related ED visits among children and youth in Ontario, Canada. *Health Affairs, 39*(10), 1728–1736H. https://doi.org/10.1377/hlthaff.2020.00232

Hill, A. J., & Jones, D. B. (2021). Self-fulfilling prophecies in the classroom. *Journal of Human Capital, 15*(3), 400–431. https://doi.org/10.1086/715204

Hoover, S., & Bostic, J. (2021). Schools as a vital component of the child and adolescent mental health system. *Psychiatric Services, 72*(1), 37–48.

Jang, E. E., & Sinclair, J. (2018). Ontario's educational assessment policy and practice: A double-edged sword? *Assessment in Education: Principles, Policy & Practice, 25*(6), 655–677. https://doi.org/10.1080/0969594X.2017.1329705

Mental Health Commission of Canada. (2021, November 25). *Children and youth.* https://mental-healthcommission.ca/what-we-do/children-and-youth/

Miles, J. (2021). Curriculum reform in a culture of redress: How social and political pressures are shaping social studies curriculum in Canada. *Journal of Curriculum Studies, 53*(1), 47–64. https://doi.org/10.1080/00220272.2020.1822920

Samuel Centre for Social Connectedness. (n.d.). *Making Indigenous-led education a public policy priority: The benefits of land-based education and programming.* https://www.socialconnect-edness.org/wp-content/uploads/2019/10/Land-Based-Education-Pamphlet.pdf

Starblanket, G., Long, D. A., & Dickason, O. P. (2020). *Visions of the heart: Issues involving indigenous peoples in Canada* (5th ed.). Oxford University Press.

Testing, Stress, and Performance: How Students Respond Physiologically to High-Stakes Testing. (2018). National Bureau of Economic Research, Inc. https://doi.org/10.3386/w25305

Vaillancourt, T., Szatmari, P., Georgiades, K., & Krygsman, A. (2021). The impact of COVID-19 on the mental health of Canadian children and youth. *Facets (Ottawa), 6*(1), 1628–1648. https://doi.org/10.1139/facets-2021-0078

# AwakenU: Exploring the Transformative Power of Meditative Inquiry in Higher Education During the COVID-19 Pandemic

**J. L. Rebek and J. M. Barone**

## Introduction

In this age of distraction and mental health issues, faculty are obligated to engage students in awareness—of themselves, their world, their learning, and their roles as future leaders. The value of connecting learners with themselves to cultivate awareness is integral to learning and has been described as meditative inquiry (MI). MI instills personal transformation as a conduit to transformational learning through critical reflexivity and dialogue—examining how one thinks, feels, and acts via meditation (Kumar, 2013). This self-awareness is critical to the field of leadership development because it transforms individuals into creatively discovering new and better ways of being and interacting with the world (Barbezat & Bush, 2014). In the context of the COVID-19 pandemic, this research explored mindfulness as a contemplative pedagogy for undergraduate well-being via an 8-week AwakenU intervention. With the prevailing mental health challenges affecting undergraduate students, the overall goal of the program was to facilitate personal development by offering participants tools to actualize their leadership potential, increase productivity, and promote experiences of meaningfulness and well-being.

Leadership is the practical process of guiding oneself (intrapersonal development) or others (interpersonal) and is open to anyone. A strong character and self-awareness are the foundation for authentic leadership, especially when driven by a genuine cause rather than ego (Mortensen et al., 2014; as cited in Rebek, 2019). Ultimately, authentic leadership is about personal choices, courage, and the commitment to make a positive impact. This study addressed the need for authentic leadership in today's labor force by examining the impact of MI within an

J. L. Rebek (✉) · J. M. Barone
School of Business and Economics, Algoma University, Sault Ste. Marie, ON, Canada
e-mail: jody.rebek@algomau.ca

intrapersonal or leader development intervention. A sequential explanatory mixed methods approach explored the impact of undergraduate students engaging in MI, considering its influence on aspects such as emotional regulation, self-esteem, self-care, creativity, and benevolence. Data collected involved psychometric scales, including the Mindful Self-Care Scale (MSCS), the Emotional Regulation Questionnaire (ERQ, measuring a tendency to regulate emotions), the Rosenberg Self-Esteem Scale (RSES, measuring positive and negative feelings about the self), and the Creative Achievement Questionnaire (CAQ, measuring achievement across ten domains of creativity). The study was conducted in a loving, joyful, and intellectually stimulating environment, acknowledging the importance of establishing a safe space for personal transformation (where people feel valued). The findings of this research aim to provide valuable insights for educational leaders and curriculum developers seeking to enhance leadership development in undergraduate students. By shedding light on the potential of MI as a pedagogical tool, this study underscores the significance of integrating contemplative practices into postsecondary education. When carefully and thoughtfully designed, MI illustrates the potential to initiate a profound learning experience for personal growth, opening self-awareness and well-being, generating the authentic approaches needed to navigate our ever-changing world.

## Literature Review

Meditation and contemplative practices have gained recognition in higher education since they are valuable tools in promoting well-being, enhancing academic performance, and fostering personal and professional growth among undergraduate students (Behan, 2020). We will summarize the history, role, and impact of mindfulness and MI in higher education on undergraduate well-being.

### *History and Benefits of Meditation in Higher Education*

Meditation is a contemplative ancient spiritual and philosophical tradition that has been found in contemporary higher education courses (e.g., Dr. Laurie Santos, Stanford). Previously, meditation was linked with religious and spiritual contexts. Practices like MI, which incorporate meditation, evolved into a focusing practice to enhance mental and emotional well-being and cognitive development (Davidson et al., 2003). Some benefits of meditation in higher education are the following:

- Lowered stress and anxiety—Many studies involving undergraduate students demonstrated the effectiveness of meditation, especially mindfulness-based meditation in reducing stress and anxiety levels among college students (Ramel et al., 2004).

- Increased focus and concentration—Meditation proved to improve attention and concentration, having a positive impact on undergraduates' academic performance due to higher levels of engagement (Rebek, 2019).
- Increased emotional regulation—Meditation promotes emotional intelligence and aids undergraduates in better managing emotions, enhancing interpersonal relations, and thus contributing to a positive classroom environment (Goleman, 2013; Rao, 2008; Senge, 2006).
- Improved cognition—Studies showed a link between meditation and improved cognitive functions such as problem-solving, memory, and creativity, which benefit undergraduates' learning (Napora, 2013).
- Enhanced well-being: Meditation also enhances a sense of well-being, self-awareness, and self-compassion and are key components of overall undergraduate well-being (Lucas & Goodman, 2015; Rae, 2015).

Faculty must establish a safe or brave space, designed with thoughtfulness and care, to integrate contemplative practices or MI meaningfully, while acknowledging the dangers and risks (Anālayo, 2021). Providing support and resources for any psychological or mental health issues is essential. Critical elements to establish a brave space include—building psychological safety, sharing vulnerability, and establishing a shared purpose to promote a sense of belonging to members (Coyle, 2018).

## *Role of Meditative Inquiry (MI) in Higher Education*

MI is a contemplative pedagogy that integrates ancient wisdom traditions of meditation into an educational context (Kumar, 2013). It emphasizes self-discovery, critical reflection, authentic leadership development, experiential learning, and personal well-being. The incorporation of MI in higher education has several notable implications:

- Encourages **self-discovery**, self-exploration, and growth: With this framework as a guide students are encouraged to explore their complex inner world, personal growth, and self-awareness. This could lead to increased adaptability, resilience, and strengthened motivation.
- Enhanced learning and **creativity**: MI promotes creative and critical thinking, encouraging students to examine thought processes and mental models. It can lead to innovative problem-solving and a deeper understanding of course material, strengthening academic performance.
- **Authentic leadership development**: MI can serve as a platform for developing authentic leadership skills, emphasizing values, ethics, and compassion. Recognizing leadership qualities requires an individual to have the courage to face oneself. "The term leader has nothing to do with position, status, or number of direct reports" (Brown, 2018, p. 185). It is all about intentions, choices made, and the bravery to show up and share. "If you want to change the way of being,

you have to change the way of doing" (Garton, 2017). Authentic, genuine and compassionate behaviours from faculty open students to feel accepted for their authenticity.

- Emotional **well-being** and interpersonal relationships: Meditation practices reduce symptoms of depression, anxiety, and stress thus contributing to emotional well-being. Meditation also fosters empathy, self-compassion, and better interpersonal communication, promoting positive relationships with peers and faculty.
- **Benevolence**: Meditation nurtures compassion and care toward self and others. Benevolence is a dimension of trustworthiness that encapsulates generosity, kindness, and overall goodness (Svare et al., 2020).

MI has the capacity to generate a "psychological revolution" that comes about through self-awareness, which rises from deep self-reflexivity—to return inward and witness self-accountability (Kumar, 2013, p. 10). Awareness or MI is not a critical engagement but rather a compassionate observation of self, to experience and witness the content of the mind, heart, and soul directly as it operates from moment to moment (Kumar, 2013).

Literature demonstrates that meditation or MI has a significant and positive impact on undergraduate well-being in higher education. As higher education institutions increasingly recognize the importance of student well-being, the integration of meditation and MI into the curriculum becomes more imperative to successful learning. Further research is needed to explore the long-term effects and best practices for implementing these contemplative practices in higher education, including differences in gender, race, and culture and between virtual and in-person differentiators.

## Methodology

Methods that focus on actualizing human potential lead to more productive, meaningful lives (Luthans & Youssef, 2004). AwakenU was initiated to engage students in well-being and leader development during the COVID-19 pandemic, in both synchronous and asynchronous formats. Participants were invited to engage in the research (informed consent). Quantitative and qualitative data were collected simultaneously but analyzed sequentially at the end of this explanatory mixed methods study (Palinkas et al., 2019). A case study approach was combined with randomized control trial (RCT; Merriam, 1998; Stake, 1995). The qualitative data collected included arts-integrated methods within the domain of Positive Organizational Scholarship (POS; Seligman, 2002). Arts-integrated inquiries infuse new life and renew the potential for transformation of participants and are often used for leadership studies (Taylor & Ladkin, 2009). Methods that focus on actualizing human potential lead to more productive, meaningful lives (Luthans & Youssef, 2004).

The following methods were also explored:

I. *Focus Group*: Participants who volunteered to participate discussed their experience and the impact of these practices on their self-awareness and life.

II. *Online Surveys*: Quantitative data was collected using the following psychometric scales: Self-care scale (Cook-Cottone & Guyker, 2018; Hotchkiss & Cook-Cottone, 2019), Emotional Regulation Questionnaire (ERQ, measuring a tendency to regulate emotions), Rosenberg Self-Esteem Scale (RSES, measuring positive and negative feelings about the self), and the Creative Achievement Questionnaire (CAQ, measuring achievement across 10 domains of creativity). Based on past research in meditation and the benefits of MI, these domains were chosen.

III. *Interviews:* Using purposeful sampling (Patton, 2005), key informant interviews were conducted to deepen knowledge.

IV. *Artifacts* (i.e., reflections, artworks, poems, etc.) were presented each week as an extension of the mindfulness prompts and were provided by participants who accepted the invitation to do so. A parallax praxis model was used to evaluate the artifacts which "has the capacity to evoke change because the arts are emotive and can powerfully re/injure or re/produce memories. Deep ethical care must be considered" (Sameshima et al., 2019, p. 55).

Due to the participation rate, some quantitative analyses could not be performed (e.g., asynchronous versus synchronous participation, color analysis, affective language codes). All qualitative data was analyzed by research assistants and principal researchers separately and then compared to strengthen the validity. Interview codes and themes (relating to questions in quantitative scales) were assigned until a point of saturation (e.g., no new codes or categories). Themes and codes were then applied to the focus group and artifact analysis. Once researchers completed their individual qualitative data analysis, they compared the codes and themes to determine any significant similarities, differences, and outliers. Based on the researchers' analysis, they refined the codes and grouped them into themes. Quantitative analysis was shared in a focus group with all researchers for input and validation of qualitative themes and codes (i.e., similar or different relationships).

# Findings

The main themes participants expressed included exploration and creativity around their self-identity and self-reflection which enhanced their self-awareness and self-esteem (feelings shifting from no good, useless, failure *to* positive attitude, respect, and pride). Participants experienced this development and growth through struggles and a journey of dichotomies. Many participants drew on positive vocabulary to describe their internal feelings, along with their self and their worldviews. Others contrasted this with dark, strong vocabulary (e.g., sorrow, tragedy, doom, morbid, daunting) to describe themselves, their feelings, and their world. Participants' efforts led to personal growth (the uncomfortable and the comfortable) and expressed more benevolence toward self and others. Participants discussed benevolence in terms of "giving others a chance" and being "deserving of kindness" and goodness. One participant experienced "compassion fatigue" due to exposure to traumatic events in the media (e.g., unmarked graves at Canadian residential schools). This historical moment served as an opportunity to engage participants in understanding Truth and Reconciliation (TRC) with First Nations and the idea of making sacrifices for the greater good of people (equity, diversity, and inclusion) and the planet in our daily decisions.

Interestingly, participants varied in their ranking of virtues before and after participating in the AwakenU intervention (which corresponded to the eight-session themes: acceptance, authenticity, benevolence, honesty, humility, joy, well-being, and wisdom). The meditation group demonstrated a lower ranking of authenticity ($z = -2.20$, $p < 0.05$) and a higher ranking of acceptance ($z = -2.12$, $p < 0.05$) among the virtues. The writing group did not have a similar shift in the perceived value of these virtues. Nonparametric Wilcoxon signed-rank tests were employed, and there were no significant changes detected in the CAQ, RSES, or ERQ subscales, including cognitive reappraisal and expression suppression ($p > 0.05$).

## Discussion/Interpretation/Conclusion

Participants engaged in self-reflection, leading to introspection, awareness, and compassionate evaluation of their perceptions. The weekly themes influenced their lives, motivating them to commit to personal growth and engaging them in applying additional coping tools (with mental health support available 24/7). Cultivating a deeper self-relationship was important for participants, and they acknowledged this process required effort, discipline, accountability, and time. Some participants experienced a shift in their perspective on mindfulness, recognizing the versatility of embracing silence, accepting, and being present to their thoughts and emotions in a real way. Participants ($n = 20$ due to attrition and data scrubbing) experienced a noteworthy shift in their perceived value of two virtues: authenticity and acceptance. This suggests that within a relatively short period (i.e., two months), perceptions can be altered to encourage personal development, potentially leading to positive outcomes for both individuals and groups.

This study contributes significantly to the understanding of the role of MI in higher education. It provides evidence of its positive impact on well-being and authentic development. The study encourages educational institutions to carefully consider incorporating contemplative practices as a means to prepare students for a complex and demanding world while fostering personal transformation. It is important to note that any introduction of contemplative practices requires serious time and effort in developing oneself. It also requires training/knowledge to understand the dangers, risks, and ways to provide compassionately introduct and provide important supports students need for such sacred work (Anālayo, 2021; Choi et al., 2021).

# References

Anālayo, B. (2021). The dangers of mindfulness: Another myth? *Mindfulness, 12*(12), 2890–2895.

Barbezat, D. P. & Bush, M. (2014). Contemplative practices in higher education: Powerful methods to transform teaching and learning. San Francisco, CA: Jossey-Bass. https://doi.org/10.1080/1360144X.2014.998876

Behan, C. (2020). The benefits of meditation and mindfulness practices during times of crisis such as COVID-19. *Irish Journal of Psychological Medicine, 37*(4), 256–258. https://doi.org/10.1007/s12671-021-01682-w

Brown, B. (2018). *Dare to lead: Brave work. Tough conversations. Whole hearts.* Random house.

Choi, E., Farb, N. A. S., Pogrebtsova, E., Gruman, J., & Grossmann, I. (2021). What do people mean when they talk about mindfulness? *Clinical Psychology Review, 89*(2012), 1–15. https://doi.org/10.1016/j.cpr.2021.102085

Cook-Cottone, C. P., & Guyker, W. M. (2018). The development and validation of the mindful self-care scale (MSCS): An assessment of practices that support positive embodiment. *Mindfulness, 9*(1), 161–175.

Coyle, D. (2018). *The culture code: The secrets of highly successful groups.* Bantam Books.

Davidson, R. J., Kabat-Zinn, J., Schumacher, J., Rosenkranz, M., Muller, D., Santorelli, S. F., Urbanowski, F., Harrington, A., Bonus, K., & Sheridan, J. F. (2003). Alterations in brain and immune function produced by mindfulness meditation. *Psychosomatic Medicine, 65*(4), 564–570. https://doi.org/10.1097/01.PSY.0000077505.67574.E3

Garton, E. (2017, April 25). How to be an inspiring leader. *Harvard Business Review.* https://hbr.org/2017/04/how-to-be-an-inspiring-leader

Goleman, D. (2013). *Focus: The hidden driver of excellence.* HarperCollins.

Hotchkiss, J. T., & Cook-Cottone, C. P. (2019). Validation of the Mindful Self-Care Scale (MSCS) and development of the brief-MSCS among hospice and healthcare professionals: A confirmatory factor analysis approach to validation. *Palliative & Supportive Care, 17*(6), 628–636.

Kumar, A. (2013). *Curriculum as meditative inquiry.* Springer.

Lucas, N., & Goodman, F. R. (2015). Well-being, leadership, and positive organizational scholarship: A case study of project-based learning in higher education. *Journal of Leadership Education, 2015*(14), 138–152. https://doi.org/10.12806/V14/I4/T2

Luthans, F., & Youssef, C. M. (2004). Human, social, and now positive psychological capital management: Investing in people for competitive advantage. *Organizational Dynamics, 33*(2), 143–160.

Merriam, S. B. (1998). *Qualitative research and case study applications in education.* Jossey-Bass.

Napora, L. (2013). *The impact of classroom-based meditation practice on cognitive engagement, mindfulness and academic performance of undergraduate college students.* Doctoral dissertation. University at Buffalo, State University of New York.

Patton, M. Q. (2005). *Qualitative research: Encyclopedia of statistics in behavioral science.* Hoboken: *NJ: John Wiley & Sons.*

Palinkas, L. A., Mendon, S. J., & Hamilton, A. B. (2019). Innovations in mixed methods evaluations. *Annual Review of Public Health, 40,* 423–442.

Rae, V. (2015). *The developing mind: A qualitative multi-case study of the intra- and interpersonal learning experiences and practices of mindfulness-based practitioners.* Doctoral dissertation, Shenandoah University. Proquest Dissertations.

Ramel, W., Goldin, P. R., Carmona, P. E., & McQuaid, J. R. (2004). The effects of mindfulness meditation on cognitive processes and affect in patients with past depression. *Cognitive Therapy and Research, 28*(4), 433–455.

Rao, S. S. (2008). The shape of leadership to come. *Business Strategy Review, 19*(1), 54–58. https://doi.org/10.1111/j.1467-8616.2008.00519.x

Rebek, J. L. (2019). *Mindful leader development of undergraduate students.* Doctoral dissertation. Retrieved from Lakehead University Knowledge Commons. https://knowledgecommons.lakeheadu.ca/handle/2453/4508

Sameshima, P., Maarhuis, P. L., & Wiebe, S. (2019). *Parallaxic praxis: Multimodal interdisciplinary pedagogical research design*. Vernon Press.

Seligman, M. E. (2002). Positive psychology, positive prevention, and positive therapy. *Handbook of Positive Psychology, 2*, 3–12.

Senge, P. M. (2006). *The fifth discipline: The art and practice of the learning organization*. Broadway Business.

Stake, R. (1995). *The art of case study research*. Sage.

Svare, H., Gausdal, A. H., & Möllering, G. (2020). The function of ability, benevolence, and integrity-based trust in innovation networks. *Industry and Innovation, 27*(6), 585–604.

Taylor, S. S., & Ladkin, D. (2009). Understanding arts-based methods in managerial development. *Academy of Management Learning & Education, 8*(1), 55–69.

# "Normal" Response to "Abnormal" Circumstances: Helping Students Thrive Post-pandemic

Teryn Bruni

## Introduction

In the wake of the global pandemic, university and college students experienced disruptions in learning, financial hardship, health-related stress, loss and grief, and the constant surge of uncertainty surrounding lockdown measures, health protocols, and academic expectations (Appleby et al., 2022; Copeland et al., 2021). Students from racialized and marginalized groups were disproportionately impacted by these challenges (Kim et al., 2022; Zimmermann et al., 2021) and were most negatively affected (Hamza et al., 2021; Son et al., 2020). Although impacts of the pandemic have been witnessed and discussed by educators across the postsecondary sector, research suggests faculty may underestimate the short- and long-term impact of the pandemic on the personal and academic lives of students (Olson et al., 2023).

As we return to pre-pandemic academic life, students continue to face significant academic and mental health challenges. Academic demands have shifted back to pre-pandemic standards, and many students have not been exposed to the learning opportunities required to succeed in this "new" academic environment. The scaffolding and skill development typically afforded within the first year of studies were not available to this group of students due to the abrupt shift to a largely virtual learning environment. Pandemic-related disruptions in learning, increased stress, and isolation among secondary school students will also have an impact on incoming first- and second-year undergraduate student success (Rao & Rao, 2021). Postsecondary institutions are now faced with an important task to provide students with the necessary support to learn and thrive within a pre-pandemic learning environment.

T. Bruni (✉)
Department of Psychology, Algoma University, Sault ste Marie, ON, Canada
e-mail: teryn.bruni@algomau.ca

Mental health is most commonly the area of focus when discussing post-COVID impacts on students (Kim et al., 2022; Son et al., 2020; Zimmermann et al., 2021). Thus, it is tempting to argue that solutions will only come from increased mental health support afforded to students through access to wellness resources, counseling support services, and the provision of formal academic accommodations. Such services are critical, and successful implementation of these supports should be carefully monitored and evaluated to ensure student mental health needs are being met. Yet, we need to be mindful of over-pathologizing students for their "normal" response to very "abnormal" circumstances brought on by the pandemic and at the same time validate their feelings of distress. This may require a shift in how we, as faculty, evaluate, teach, and mentor students within and outside the classroom.

The integration of academic skill development into the curriculum, the universal provision of strategies that promote psychological flexibility (Katajavuori et al., 2023; Yao et al., 2023), and increased student access to faculty mentorship has the potential to build resilience among our students and help them be successful. Faculty are in a unique position to champion innovative approaches to better support student learning and well-being. As educators we have a responsibility to meet students where they are and to adapt expectations in a manner that not only normalizes the challenges students have faced over the last 3 years but also acknowledges the collective and unique challenges many students continue to face.

# References

Appleby, J. A., King, N., Saunders, K. E., Bast, A., Rivera, D., Byun, J., Cunningham, S., Khera, C., & Duffy, A. C. (2022). Impact of the COVID-19 pandemic on the experience and mental health of university students studying in Canada and the UK: A cross-sectional study. *BMJ Open, 12*(1), e050187. https://doi.org/10.1136/BMJOPEN-2021-050187

Copeland, W. E., McGinnis, E., Bai, Y., Adams, Z., Nardone, H., Devadanam, V., Rettew, J., & Hudziak, J. J. (2021). Impact of COVID-19 pandemic on college student mental health and wellness. *Journal of the American Academy of Child & Adolescent Psychiatry, 60*(1), 134–141. e2. https://doi.org/10.1016/J.JAAC.2020.08.466

Hamza, C. A., Ewing, L., Heath, N. L., & Goldstein, A. L. (2021). When social isolation is nothing new: A longitudinal study on psychological distress during COVID-19 among university students with and without preexisting mental health concerns. *Canadian Psychology, 62*(1), 20–30. https://doi.org/10.1037/CAP0000255

Katajavuori, N., Vehkalahti, K., & Asikainen, H. (2023). Promoting university students' well-being and studying with an acceptance and commitment therapy (ACT)-based intervention. *Current Psychology, 42*(6), 4900–4912. https://doi.org/10.1007/S12144-021-01837-X/TABLES/4

Kim, H., Rackoff, G. N., Fitzsimmons-Craft, E. E., Shin, K. E., Zainal, N. H., Schwob, J. T., Eisenberg, D., Wilfley, D. E., Taylor, C. B., & Newman, M. G. (2022). College mental health before and during the COVID-19 pandemic: Results from a nationwide survey. *Cognitive Therapy and Research, 46*(1), 1–10. https://doi.org/10.1007/S10608-021-10241-5/TABLES/3

Olson, R., Fryz, R., Essemiah, J., Crawford, M., King, A., & Fateye, B. (2023). Mental health impacts of COVID-19 lockdown on US college students: Results of a photoelicitation project. *Journal of American College Health, 71*(2), 411–421. https://doi.org/10.1080/07448481.202 1.1891921/SUPPL_FILE/VACH_A_1891921_SM3621.DOCX

Rao, M. E., & Rao, D. M. (2021). The mental health of high school students during the COVID-19 pandemic. *Frontiers in Education, 6,* 719539. https://doi.org/10.3389/FEDUC.2021.719539/BIBTEX

Son, C., Hegde, S., Smith, A., Wang, X., & Sasangohar, F. (2020). Effects of COVID-19 on college students' mental health in the United States: Interview survey study. *Journal of Medical Internet Research, 22*(9), E21279. https://www.jmir.org/2020/9/E21279. https://doi.org/10.2196/21279

Yao, X., Xu, X., Chan, K. L., Chen, S., Assink, M., & Gao, S. (2023). Associations between psychological inflexibility and mental health problems during the COVID-19 pandemic: A three-level meta-analytic review. *Journal of Affective Disorders, 320,* 148–160. https://doi.org/10.1016/J.JAD.2022.09.116

Zimmermann, M., Bledsoe, C., & Papa, A. (2021). Initial impact of the COVID-19 pandemic on college student mental health: A longitudinal examination of risk and protective factors. *Psychiatry Research, 305,* 114254. https://doi.org/10.1016/J.PSYCHRES.2021.114254

# Diasporic Queer and Trans Filipinos in Canada: Some Considerations for Anti-oppressive Mental Healthcare Practice

Fritz Pino

## Literature Review

As a trans Filipino woman, my worries and anxieties during the pandemic went beyond Canadian national borders. I worried about the survival of my queer and trans friends and their families who are in the Philippines where the healthcare system had been overwhelmed and became more inaccessible. I worried about the increased family tensions and conflicts that diasporic queer and trans Filipinos experience if they fail to send remittance to their families in the Philippines and that may result in exacerbated forms of homophobia and transphobia from their own families. In the midst of this, I find solace in thinking about the ways in which queer and trans Filipinos in the diaspora find ways to cope, such as by engaging in spirituality especially when dealing with death and loss during the pandemic.

I opened with this personal lived experience to contextualize the literature that resonates with this experience. I highlight here Martin Manalansan's (2003) work on Filipino gay men in the diaspora. Manalansan described how queer Filipinos continued to identify with the cultural script of the "bakla" while being in the diaspora. "Bakla" is not necessarily a direct translation of North American, Western conceptualization of queerness. Rather, the "bakla" identity is embedded with Filipino queer cultural sexual practices in the Philippines. For example, in terms of sexual intimacy, the bakla is attracted to and develops sexual relationship with cisgender Filipino men. In this relationship dynamics, the customary practice is that the "bakla" is expected to provide financial resources to the cisgender man or

F. Pino (✉)
University of Regina, Regina, SK, Canada
e-mail: fritz.pino@uregina.ca

"lalake" to make the relationship work (Manalansan, 2003; Pino, 2017). Many queer and trans Filipinos in the diaspora, especially those who were born and raised in the Philippines and have engaged in this queer practice, continue to carry and identify with this bakla sexual intimacy script in Canada (e.g., see Pino, 2017).

Another important feature is that diasporic queer and trans Filipinos whose direct family members (e.g., parents, siblings, relatives) are living in the Philippines, send remittance to financially support them. Many of my chosen families and relatives who lost their jobs in Canada during the pandemic struggled to fulfill this role. In my dissertation, I described how this act of sending remittance by older Filipino gay men is a form of care for their families who were left in the Philippines, as well as their way of negotiating heteronormative expectations from such families of origin (Pino, 2019b).

Speaking of spirituality, which I included in my personal observation, I noted in my previous publication the notion of "emotional contradiction" that diasporic queer and trans Filipinos experience when they get to engage with the mainstream religion (i.e., Catholicism) to experience a sense of spirituality (Pino, 2019a). Using my own transnational personal autobiographical account and drawing from postcolonial theory, emotional contradiction means having multiple, ambivalent feelings along with one's spiritual experience. This is because of how dominant religious doctrines via the priests' homily in the Philippines continue to discriminate queer and trans Filipinos, rendering their practices as "wrong." Emotional contradiction signifies the sense of agency of queer and trans Filipinos as they see both the possibilities and limits when engaging with dominant religion (Pino, 2019a).

Given these scenarios and context, I asked: how can we be thoughtful and mindful of these transnational connections and cultural nuances and scripts when considering an anti-oppressive approach to mental healthcare for diasporic queer and trans Filipinos? How do we give room for these diasporic and cultural scripts of queerness to be narrated fully by queer and trans Filipinos within a therapeutic context?

I thought of my previous publication on anti-racist and anti-oppressive mental healthcare practice framework (Ocampo & Pino, 2014). In it, together with my co-author, we discussed how mental health scholars and activists, those who are informed by anti-racism and anti-oppressive frameworks, push for a more holistic and culturally grounded mental healthcare to address the harm and pathologization that the biomedical model has made toward historically marginalized communities (Ocampo & Pino, 2014; Fernando, 2010; Ticar & Edwards, 2022). We argued that anti-oppressive mental healthcare grounded in anti-racism disrupts the hegemony and imperialism of positivist and individualist epistemologies of Western mental healthcare and interventions (Ocampo & Pino, 2014).

However, I want to boost the significance of such anti-racist and anti-oppressive mental healthcare approach. In doing so, I suggest that such an anti-oppressive approach be more attentive to the transnational subjectivities, realities, and connections, including those of diasporic queer and trans Filipinos. Indeed, this idea of the "transnational" was not fully articulated in the previous framework (see Ocampo & Pino, 2014). By highlighting the transnational subjectivities and positionalities of diasporic queer and trans Filipinos, anti-oppressive mental healthcare further disrupts the dominant framework that universalizes Western biomedical epistemologies. In this way, we can continue to resist the pathologization of queer cultural practices deemed to fall outside of Western framework. Since the COVID-19 pandemic intensified the already existing inequalities and inequities of historically marginalized communities, an anti-oppressive mental healthcare approach attentive to the transnational realities of diasporic queers and trans would offer a more expansive understanding of this community.

## Methodology

I juxtapose my personal lived experiences as a trans Filipino woman during the pandemic with the limitations of the dominant Western mental healthcare that failed to fully acknowledge diverse cultural practices and epistemologies of queerness and transness. This allowed me to invoke the anti-racist and anti-oppressive frameworks (see Ocampo & Pino, 2014) that advocated for a holistic framework and interrogated the limits of Western biomedical model of mental healthcare. By reflecting on this anti-oppressive framework, I consider the transnational realities to be paid more attention by this framework. Therefore, this process of juxtaposition subsequently enhanced the resistant practices of the anti-oppressive framework, disrupting the imperial and colonial imperatives of Western individualist mental healthcare model. These critical reflective processes and reading are consistent with feminist, anti-racist, and decolonial praxis.

## Findings and Discussion

Therefore, based on this juxtaposition and critical reflection, it is important to consider the value of having a genuine understanding of queer and trans Filipinos' transnational epistemologies of queerness and transness when implementing a more anti-oppressive approach to mental healthcare. As well, validating queer and trans stories in terms of how they navigate the impact of hetero and cis normativities in places where they assert belonging such as with their families and communities is another important consideration. By doing so, we are opening up space where they can articulate their forms of resistance against the norms, stereotypes, and stigma, including stigma from in their own community and religion. Indeed, the stigma that is being resisted is not just around mental health issues but also the perception of "always already a pathological subject" because of being queer and trans.

## Implications for Practice

Having a genuine understanding of queer and trans Filipinos' transnational epistemologies of queerness and transness, including validating queer and trans stories
around how they navigate the impact of hetero and cis normativities, can serve as
ingredients to build therapeutic alliances with diasporic queer and trans Filipinos
during formal counseling sessions. While more research is needed to build knowledge and evidence from these insights, counselors, psychotherapists, and mental
health workers can engage in an anti-oppressive approach when working with diasporic queer and trans Filipinos by rethinking their use of dominant therapeutic
models grounded in individualism, which could easily erase and pathologize diasporic queer and trans Filipinos subjectivities and worldviews.

## Conclusion

Diasporic queer and trans Filipinos are faced with stigma and stereotypes related to
their sexuality, gender, and race prior to conversations around mental health and the
pandemic. These stigma and stereotypes exist both from the Filipino community
and from mainstream society.

Indeed, anti-oppressive mental healthcare has been mobilized to address these
stigma, stereotypes, and pathological points of view. However, such an anti-
oppressive framework can be enhanced even more by considering transnational cultural scripts that queer and trans Filipinos continue to identify with.

## References

Fernando, S. (2010). *Mental health, race, and culture*. Palgrave Macmillan.
Manalansan, M. F., IV. (2003). *Global divas: Filipino gay men in the diaspora*. Duke University
    Press Books.
Ocampo, M., & Pino, F. L. (2014). An anti-racism and anti-oppression framework in mental health
    practice. In R. Moodley & M. Ocampo (Eds.), *Critical psychiatry and mental health: Exploring
    the work of Suman Fernando in clinical practice* (pp. 145–155). Routledge.
Pino, F. L. (2017). Older Filipino gay men in Canada: Bridging queer theory and gerontology in
    Filipino-Canadian studies. In R. Diaz, M. Largo, & F. Pino (Eds.), *Diasporic intimacies: Queer
    Filipinos and Canadian imaginaries* (pp. 163–181). Northwestern University Press.
Pino, F. L. (2019a). Emotional contradictions: Queer Filipinos' religious and spiritual engage-
    ments in the diaspora. In N. Wane, R. A. Torres, & D. Nyaga (Eds.), *Transversing and trans-
    locatingspiritualities: Epistemological and pedagogical conversations* (pp. 149–159). Nsemia
    Publishers.
Pino, F. L. (2019b). *A different shade of grey: Intimacies of older Filipino gay men in
    Canada*. Doctoral dissertation. University of Toronto. https://tspace.library.utoronto.ca/
    handle/1807/106798
Ticar, J. E., & Edwards, F. (2022). Toward holistic and community-based interventions in the
    mental health of Black and Filipino youth. *Intersectionalities: A Global Journal of Social Work
    Analysis, Research, Policy, and Practice, 10*(1), 52–68.

# Mental Health and Social Support Among Immigrant Women in Canada: An Arts-Based Study

Maryam Motia

## Introduction

Canada is a destination for a growing number of immigrants, including immigrant women. Statistics Canada reports declination in the mental health status of immigrants due to stress and challenges for resettlement. Mental health decrement has been found more among immigrant women, compared to immigrant men, given the intersection of immigration status and gender.

Evidence suggests that social support may protect the mental health of immigrant women in Canada. In addition, engagement with art may positively impact their mental health. Creating artwork and exchanging social support may occur concurrently in community art programs (CAP) with promising psychological effects on participants. Reports on grassroots arts projects in Canada suggest similar desired consequences. Yet, there are relatively scarce Canadian-based studies in this field. My (ongoing) doctoral research project addresses this gap, exploring (A) How do immigrant women in Canada conceptualize their mental health in the context of their migratory journeys? and (B) How does art, as a research method, allow immigrant women to express their mental health experiences related to migration? Using the constructivist grounded theory, I employ a combination of arts-based research methodologies and in-depth interviews.

In this paper, consistent with my presentation at the International Conference on Mental Health and Addictions, I share the findings of the first participant I collected data with and the implications for practitioners and policymakers.

M. Motia (✉)
Wilfrid Laurier University, Waterloo, ON, Canada
e-mail: mmotia@wlu.ca

D. Nyaga, R. A. Torres (eds.), *Reimagining Mental Health and Addiction Under the Covid-19 Pandemic,* Volume 1, Advances in Mental Health and Addiction, https://doi.org/10.1007/978-3-031-58367-4_11

## Literature Review

Migration can potentially be a stressful process that may negatively impact the mental health of immigrant women (Dela Cruz et al., 2023; Koh, 2018). Social support, however, may protect their mental health (Turin et al., 2020; Zou et al., 2021). Engagement with art may also have positive effects on the mental health of these women (Clini et al., 2019; Hanania, 2018). The promising impacts of social support and artmaking may be magnified when occurring simultaneously in the form of CAP where immigrant women create artworks and exchange support at the same time (Jo et al., 2018; Rose et al., 2018).

## Methodology

In my doctoral research study, using constructivist grounded theory (Charmaz, 2006, 2014), I aim to develop a theory that explains how diverse factors, such as gender, race, class, and immigration status, may contribute to the mental health of immigrant women in Canada.

The stages of the research include a brief introduction session (half an hour), three weekly scrapbooking sessions (1.5–2 h each), and an individual interview afterward (1–1.5 h). The entire process is virtual over Zoom.

## Findings and Discussion

Although constructivist grounded theory emphasizes representing multiple voices (Clarke, 2011), to be consistent with my presentation at the conference, I share the findings related to my first research participant I refer to as P1 hereafter.

P1 was born in India, moved to Dubai when she was 6 months old, and immigrated to Canada at the age of 15 years old. P1 is 26 years old and lives in Calgary. She obtained her master's degree and worked in Public Health for the past few years. She will move to San Francisco to join her fiancé who is currently living in San Jose.

Analyzing the collected data with this participant, I developed several themes. In this paper, following my presentation at the conference, I discuss two themes: "Sense of Home" and "Availability of Support" in the following sections.

### *Sense of Home*

This theme was developed based on data from three scrapbooking sessions and P1's scrapbook. She illustrated her understanding and experiences of a feeling of belonging and a sense of home (Picture 1).

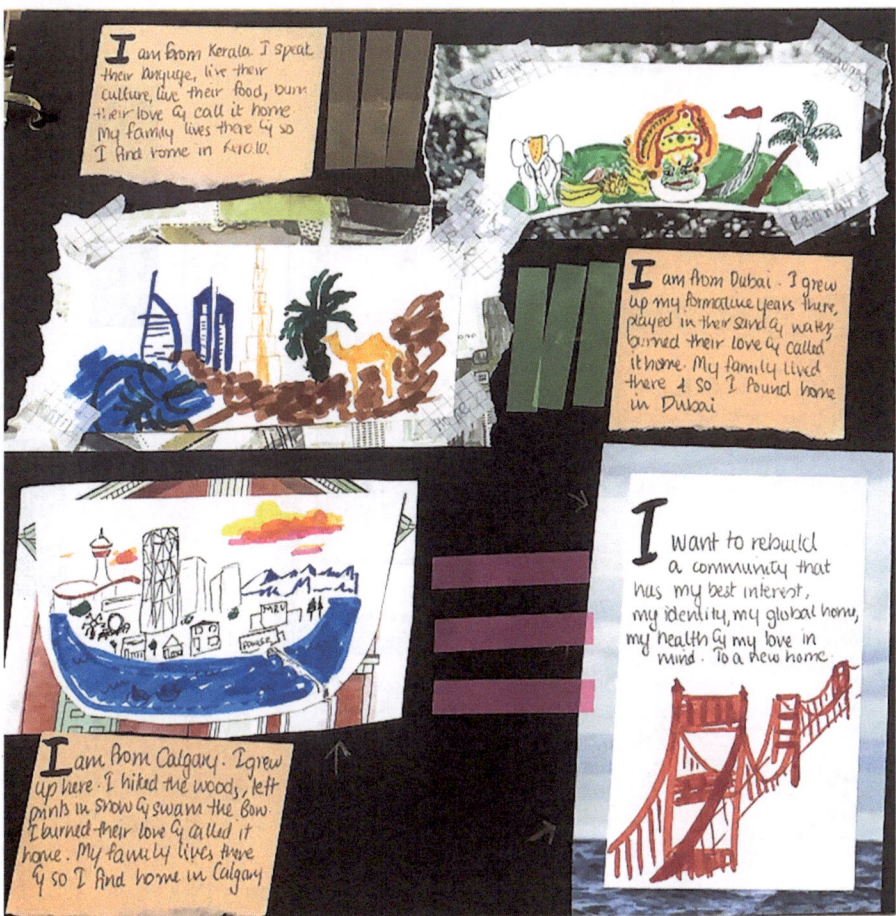

**Picture 1** "Sense of Home"

She used the tickets (Picture 2) she had bought to visit her fiancé in San Francisco and San Jose. She also used two photos reflecting her experiences of those trips and a piece of a wrap of a chocolate bar representing the Golden Gate Bridge.

The colorful pieces of the paper demonstrate her various identities contributing to her experiences of belonging and home as follows:

From the top left to the bottom left: "student," followed by "employee," "volunteer," and "explorer." She added her identities grounded in "gender" as follows: from the top right to the bottom right, "woman," followed by "daughter," "sister," and "friend."

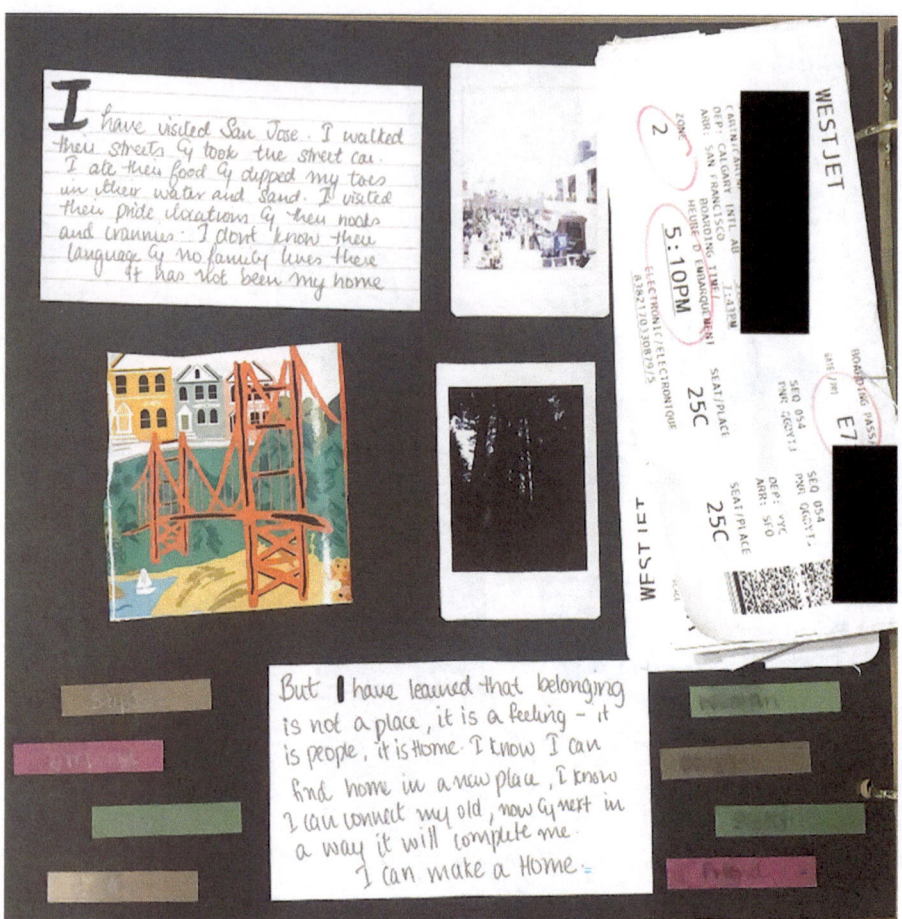

**Picture 2** "Sense of Home"

## *Availability of Support*

This theme was developed based on data collected from the scrapbooking sessions, the scrapbook, and the final interview. The house with cuts (Picture 3) shows that discussing topics related to mental health or mental health issues is forbidden at P1's place, especially with her parents. However, other family members and friends are always available to turn to, and they respond: "I understand; let me help; there's no shame." The availability and diversity of support have been illustrated on this page. The findings also reflect on the importance of "substitute" resources of support. For example, when there is no or limited support from a particular resource(s), other resources may compensate and facilitate meeting ends.

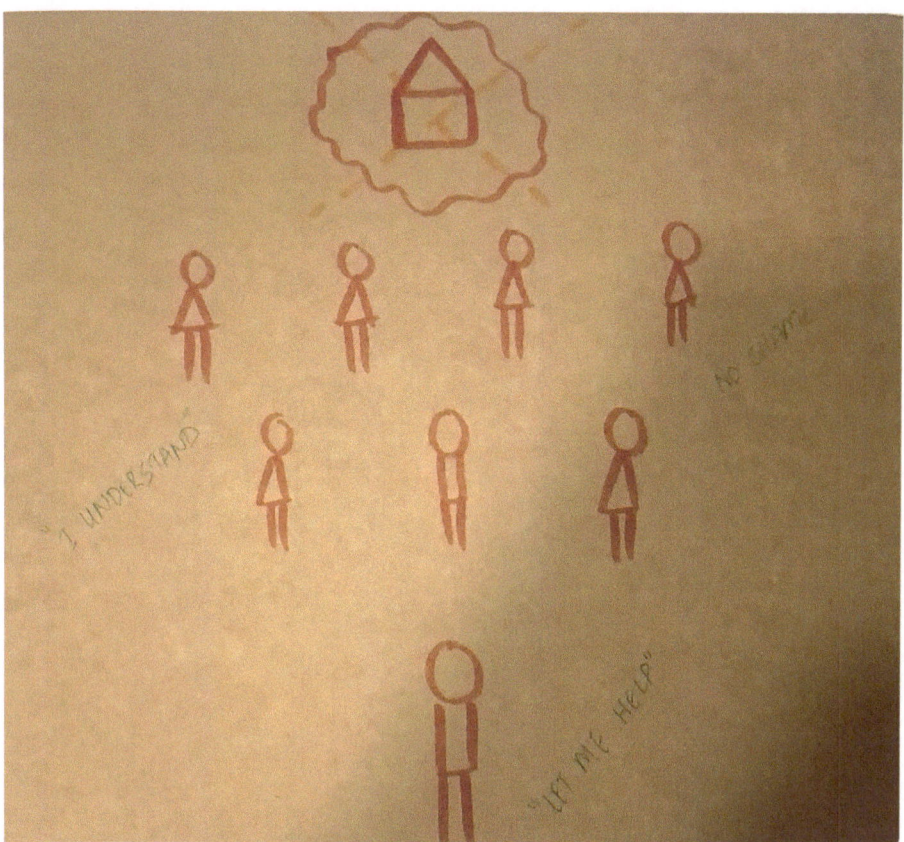

**Picture 3** "Availability of Support"

P1 demonstrates her understanding and experiences of social support through the lens of gender (Picture 4). She refers to her diverse support resources (e.g., family or professional help).

Using radar-like lines, she shows the frequency and strength of reaching out to those supportive network members. In this light, unlike professional help, friends would be the most enriched resources for her to turn to frequently.

P1 also reflects on the different types of support (e.g., informational or emotional) she receives from various resources.

The two upside-down chairs reflect her viewpoint on social support. As she states, social support is "just being there [for the other person], regardless of how the other person is at the same time." This statement reflects the importance of accountability of support resources and refers to the concept of perceived support.

In her final interview, P1 also reflects on her understanding of social support: "... for me, social support can be anyone that I find who supports me in that instant. I think it doesn't have to be a committed relationship with the friend or a partner or a family."

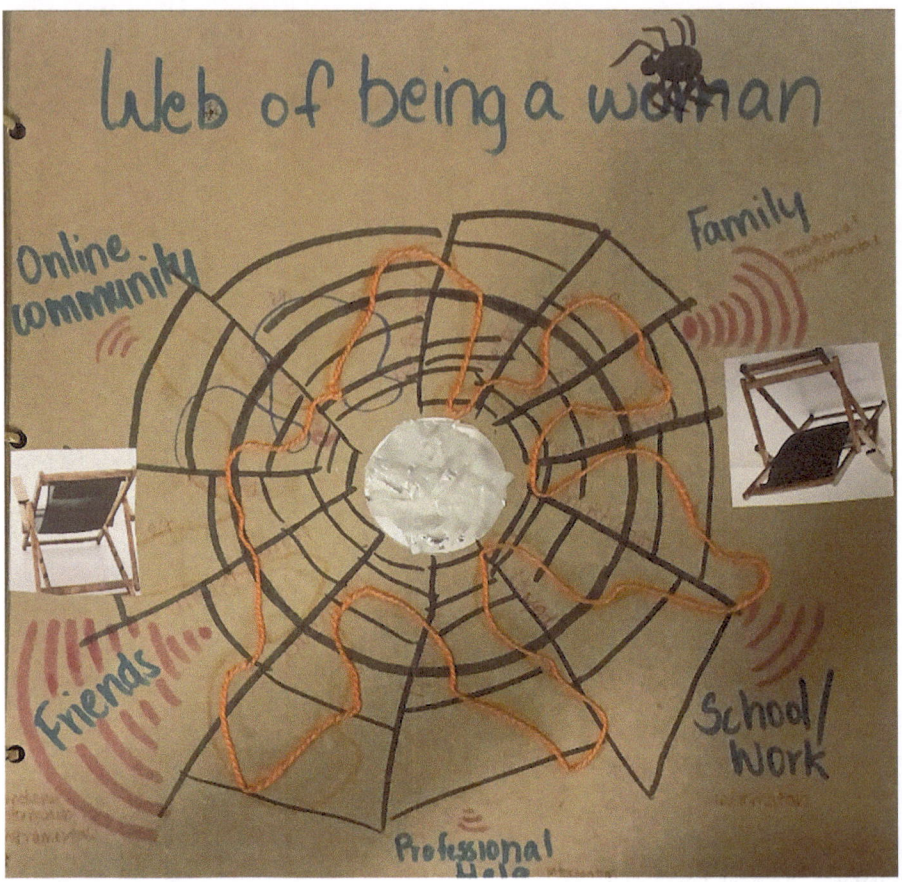

**Picture 4** "Availability of Support"

Overall, this theme highlights the significance of the quality and quantity of social support from diverse resources. It also reflects that the conceptualization of social support directly determines reaching out to and potentially receiving support from varied resources. As P1 illustrates, for her, social support means "just being there" for another person (Picture 4); she expanded on her definition of social support in the final interview as help from anyone in a given situation. These all refer to the *spontaneity* of support and the *flexibility* of support resource(s) as she views it. Both Pictures 3 and 4 demonstrating assistance she would receive from her extensive repertoire of support reflect how she conceptualizes social support and support resources as spontaneous and flexible.

The findings of this case study and preliminary findings of the main study reflect three main aspects of group scrapbooking as a space for exploring and expressing oneself, practicing previously learned skills, and exchanging social support.

# References

Charmaz, K. (2006). *Constructing grounded theory: A practical guide through qualitative analysis*. Sage Publications.

Charmaz, K. (2014). *Constructing grounded theory* (2nd ed.). Sage Publications.

Clarke, A. E. (2011). Doing situational maps and analysis. In *Situational analysis: Grounded theory after the tostmodern turn* (pp. 83–144). Sage Publications.

Clini, C., Thomson, L. J. M., & Chatterjee, H. J. (2019). Assessing the impact of artistic and cultural activities on the health and well-being of forcibly displaced people using participatory action research. *BMJ Open, 9*(e025465), 1–9. https://doi.org/10.1136/bmjopen-2018-025465

Dela Cruz, G. A., Johnstone, S., Singla, D. R., George, T. P., & Castle, D. J. (2023). A qualitative systematic review of experiences and barriers faced by migrant women with perinatal depression in Canada. *Women, 3*, 1–21. https://doi.org/10.3390/women3010001

Hanania, A. (2018). A proposal for culturally informed art therapy with Syrian refugee women: The potential for trauma expression through embroidery. *Canadian Art Therapy Association Journal, 31*(1), 33–42. https://doi.org/10.1080/08322473.2017.1378516

Jo, E., Jo, J. S., Veblen, K. K., & Potter, P. J. (2018). Enoch Senior's College for Korean immigrant seniors: Quality of life effects. *Canadian Journal on Aging/La Revue canadienne du vieillissement, 37*(3), 345–359. https://doi.org/10.1017/S0714980818000211

Koh, E. (2018). Prevalence and predictors of depression and anxiety among Korean Americans. *Social Work in Public Health, 33*(1), 55–69. https://doi.org/10.1080/19371918.2017.1415178

Rose, E., Bingley, A., Rioseco, M., & Lamb, K. (2018). Art of recovery: Displacement, mental health, and wellbeing. *Arts, 7*(94). https://doi.org/10.3390/arts7040094

Turin, T., Rashid, R., Ferdous, M., Chowdhury, N., Naeem, I., Rumana, N., Rahman, A., Rahman, N., & Lasker, M. (2020). Perceived challenges and unmet primary care access needs among Bangladeshi immigrant women in Canada. *Journal of Primary Care & Community Health, 11*, 1–10. https://doi.org/10.1177/2150132720952618

Zou, P., Shao, J., Luo, Y., Thayaparan, A., Zhang, H., Alam, A., Liu, L., & Sidani, S. (2021). Facilitators and barriers to healthy midlife transition among South Asian immigrant women in Canada: A qualitative exploration. *Healthcare, 9*(182). https://doi.org/10.3390/healthcare9020182

## *Exploring and Expressing Oneself*

Sharing scrapbooks and relevant stories and experiences would lead to learning about different experiences and viewpoints despite the similarity between the participants as immigrant women. As P1 indicates: "I really enjoyed listening to everyone's experiences, … we're all immigrant women, but the way we brought up has an immense difference in how we view things. So, it's really interesting to hear and learn from a lot of different demand on their experiences and mental health and immigration."

## *Practicing Previously Learned Skills*

As P1's scrapbook pages show, she used her skills in drawing and painting to illustrate her migratory-related experiences. Other participants also used their skills in writing and poetry when scrapbooking. The use of artistic skills that participants have already developed in their current art projects is consistent with the relevant literature.

## *Exchanging Social Support*

I observed the exchange of support within the scrapbooking groups. For instance, in one group, a more established immigrant provided informational support for the newcomer ones on how to use the healthcare system or search for jobs by developing their networks. In another group, an established immigrant who was a single mother requested me to put her in contact with a newcomer single mother to offer support in various ways.

## Conclusion

This case study indicates the richness of scrapbooking as an arts-based research method when investigating the mental health of immigrant women in Canada. The findings regarding the theme "Sense of Home" illuminate that engagement with family, community, workplace, and nature via language, food, and culture would develop a holistic view of self and foster a feeling of belonging to call a place home. The findings related to "Availability of Support" highlight the importance of conceptualization of social support on whom to turn to, support resources, and what to receive, quality and quantity of support.

# Index

© The Editor(s) (if applicable) and The Author(s), under exclusive license to                91
Springer Nature Switzerland AG 2024
D. Nyaga, R. A. Torres (eds.), *Reimagining Mental Health and Addiction Under
the Covid-19 Pandemic,* Volume 1, Advances in Mental Health and Addiction,
https://doi.org/10.1007/978-3-031-58367-4